ABANDONED
ASYLUMS OF
THE NORTHEAST

D1293814

ABANDONED
ASYLUMS OF
THE NORTHEAST

RUSTY TAGLIARENI AND
CHRISTINA MATHEWS

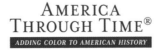

AMERICA
THROUGH TIME®
ADDING COLOR TO AMERICAN HISTORY

America Through Time is an imprint of Fonthill Media LLC
www.through-time.com
office@through-time.com

Published by Arcadia Publishing by arrangement with Fonthill Media LLC
For all general information, please contact Arcadia Publishing:
Telephone: 843-853-2070
Fax: 843-853-0044
E-mail: sales@arcadiapublishing.com
For customer service and orders:
Toll-Free 1-888-313-2665

www.arcadiapublishing.com

First published 2019

ISBN 978-1-63499-099-8

Typeset in Trade Gothic 10pt on 15pt
Printed and bound in England

CONTENTS

INTRODUCTION

For well over a decade, we have been traveling the country documenting abandoned locations—places of often great significance that, by some series of events, have fallen through the cracks. These places exist as castoffs—relics of some bygone purpose—and though perhaps forgotten by the greater world, once abandoned, these buildings take on another life, unique to their newfound solitude. Make no mistake though, the pages of this book do not celebrate death, rather life forgotten, and what comes thereafter.

The focus with this book is upon abandoned asylums. Psychiatric hospitals are a gripping subject matter in and of themselves, even while still in operation, and their histories often weave a tale that is much broader than that of the buildings themselves. Now these once-clamoring campuses are left abandoned, hushed, in grey light. There are no patients here, no doctors or nurses. All is quiet and all is dark, and in this darkness, there is peace found in reflection. As the ivy wraps the walls, there is an intense beauty here enveloped in misery.

Abandoned asylums are mysterious entities, ones that captivate the imagination and manifest their own stories without speaking a single word. Though film and television often portray these places as frightening things, these sprawling campuses were anything but that when first created. In many cases, the passion of purpose and attention to architectural detail is still visible on these structures today, though often physically obscured by peeling paint and overgrowth, and concealed in a much less tangible way by stigmas and societal perception.

It is our sincere hope that that the pages that follow may serve to celebrate the ephemeral beauty of these forsaken American institutions, while at the same time help to dispel some of the shame that plagues not only these buildings, but our modern mental healthcare system. Sometimes all one needs to better understand complex and emotionally-charged topics is a different perspective. We hope to help in providing that.

Rusty Tagliareni and Christina Mathews
www.AntiquityEchoes.com

1

PENNHURST STATE SCHOOL AND HOSPITAL

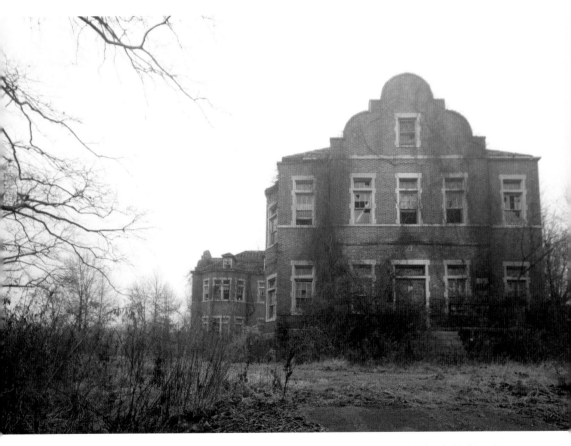

Perhaps the best way in which to introduce the former Pennhurst State School and Hospital is through a single quotation from the 1968 documentary *Suffer the Little Children*, an exposé by Bill Baldini, which focused upon the deplorable conditions under which the asylum operated. When one patient was asked by the interviewer what he would like most in the world, if he could have anything he could imagine, a sad and withdrawn reply simply stated: "To get out of Pennhurst."

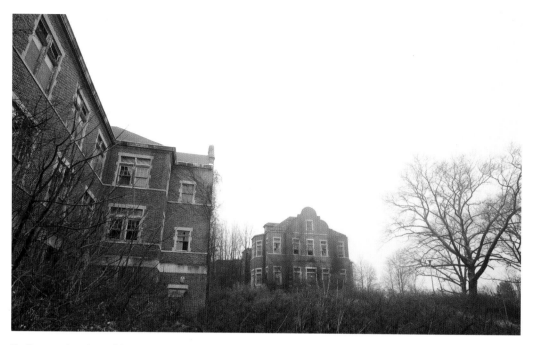

On the morning of our visit, a chilled fog hung thickly about the campus, creating a veil of gray that swallowed distant forms into vague soft-edged silhouettes, and completely concealed the sky above. The Pennhurst property had disconnected from the greater world around it, surrounded on all sides by massive walls of rolling white. It sat alone in a depressing haze. When considering the innumerable acts of cruelty and neglect that had played out here through the facility's seventy-nine years of operation, perhaps there exists no more suiting an atmosphere in which to witness these grounds.

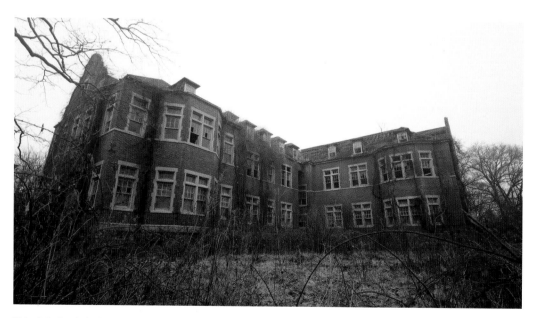

This state-funded school and hospital center was at the heart of the human rights movement that revolutionized our nation's approach to healthcare for the mentally and physically handicapped, and by extension, our views on the value of human life. Pennhurst was one of the most striking examples of the maltreatment that was characteristic of such institutions—at one point, news outlets had labeled it the "Shame of the Nation."

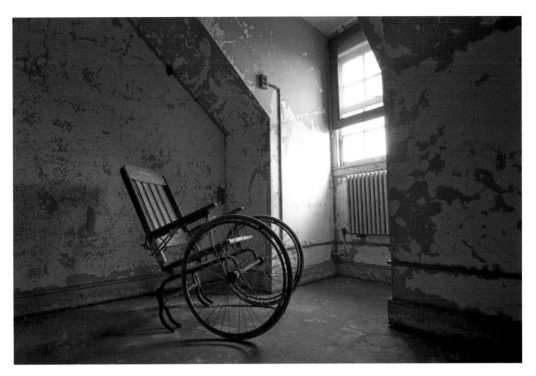

An antique wheelchair forever stares out of a window on the upper-most floor of a ward. Like the asylum building themselves, the relics left within silently reveal their stories.

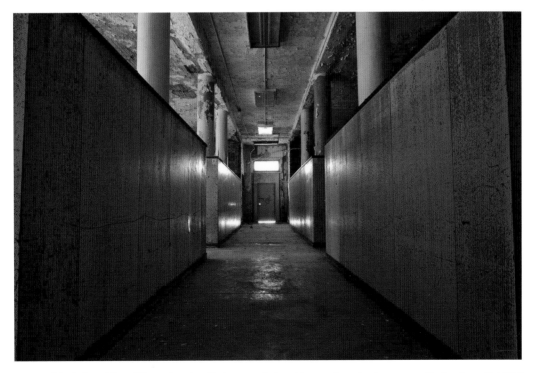

A typical ward floor at the asylum. Lengthwise, a central corridor runs through a large room of half-walls, segmenting the area into compartment-like living quarters containing several beds, small shared dressers, and little else.

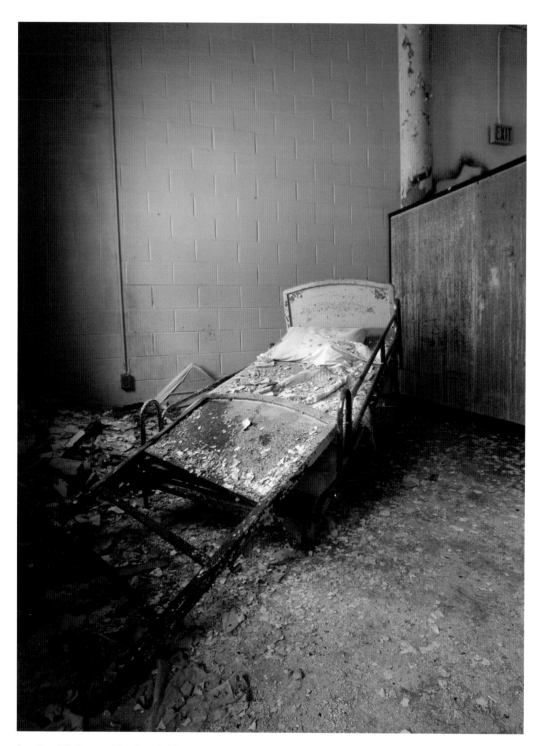

Pennhurst first opened its doors in November 1908, and due to pressure to accept not only the mentally and physically handicapped, but also immigrants, criminals, and orphans who could not be housed elsewhere, it was overcrowded within only a few years. In 1913, the "Commission for the Care of the Feeble-Minded" was appointed by Pennsylvania state legislature, and brazenly stated that those with disabilities were "unfit for citizenship" and furthermore "posed a menace to the peace."

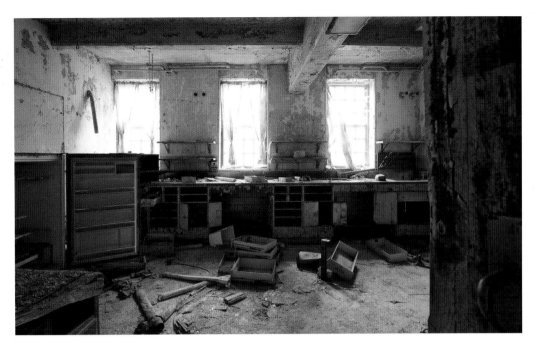

A long-disused ward pantry slowly crumbles away. Like many similar facilities of the era, Pennhurst was wholly independent from the outside world. It operated its own power plant, policed its own grounds, and grew its own food. Any additional needs were supplied by a railway, which connected to the campus. The facility could operate without any interaction with the community, and that was seemingly the way the community preferred it.

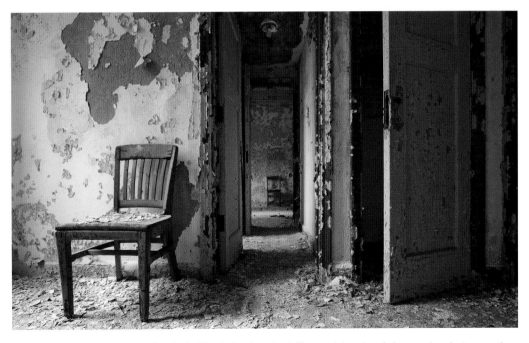

Eventually, the overcrowding, lack of funds, inadequate staffing, and decades of abuse and neglect accusations caught up with the asylum, and in 1987, Pennhurst closed its doors for good. The death of the campus was not without positive impact, though; the martyrdom of its long-suffering patients helped put into motion dramatic changes to medical practices across the country.

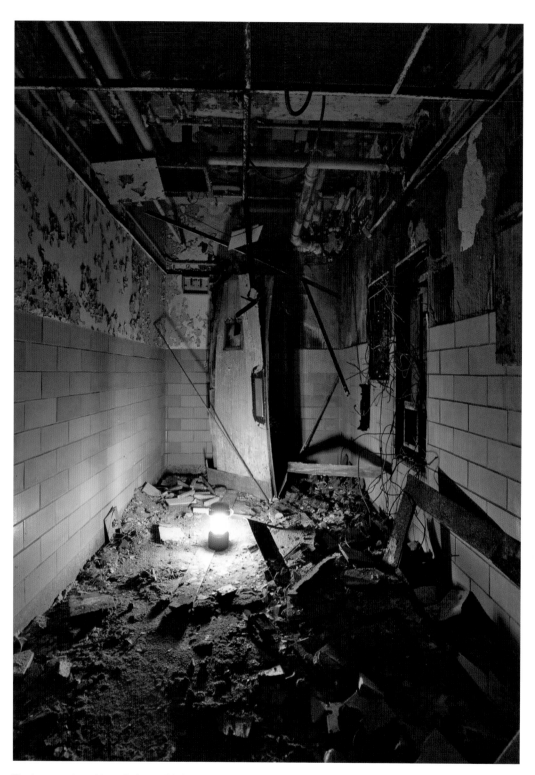

The basements and tunnels that reside below the old hospital were pitch black, and often we had to turn to our electric lantern to light the scenes before us. In this case, it was to better see the ragged doorway that we had just barely managed to pass through.

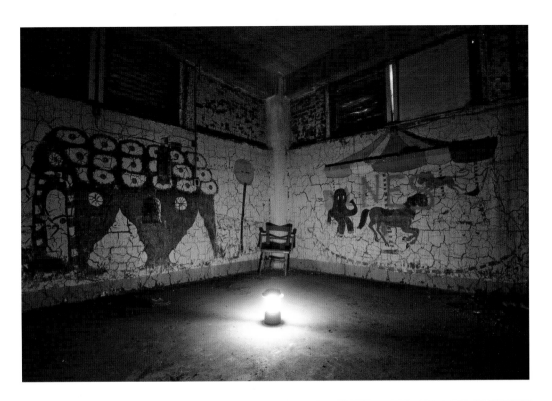

Above: The basement walls of certain buildings were painted in bright murals depicting lighthearted scenes of children playing, merry-go-rounds, and candy cottages. However, time has not treated these paintings well. Looking upon them now, knowing the somber history that took place here, the once-cheerful wall decor has come to take on a much more sinister air.

Right: In the murk and silence of the basement, you find yourself wondering not what the characters depicted on the walls are doing, but rather what horrors they may have borne witness to in their time.

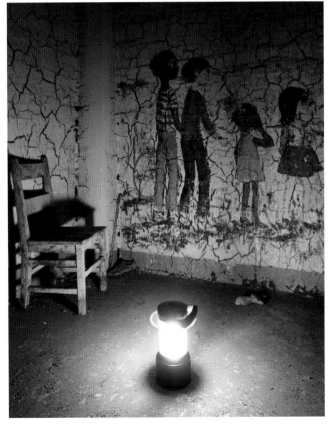

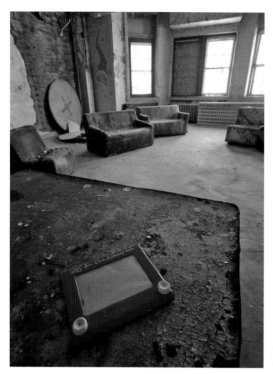

Accounts of the abuse and neglect endured by patients at overcrowded hospital centers such as Pennhurst can often be sickening. Many who resided here were abandoned by all who knew them, as forlorn as this facility itself would come to be decades later.

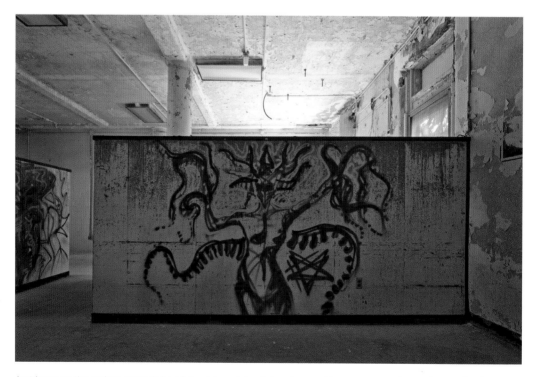

Just because the asylum grounds had fallen into a state of abandonment for many years does not mean that it was devoid of life. For quite some time, the old asylum had become a popular hangout for youths and curiosity seekers of all kinds. Many of their marks remain to this day, in the form of simple names scrawled upon the walls of the tunnels and in large-scale paintings, such as this one, on the wall of a ward bedroom.

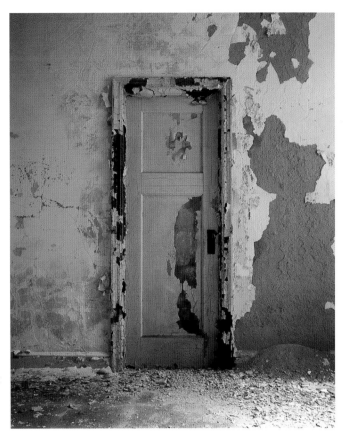

Patients at Pennhurst were grouped into several general categories, with titles that, by the standards of today, seem nearly unbelievable. Under the classification of mental prowess, one was listed as either an "imbecile" or "insane." Physically, the patient could be declared either "epileptic" or "healthy"—there existed no in-between.

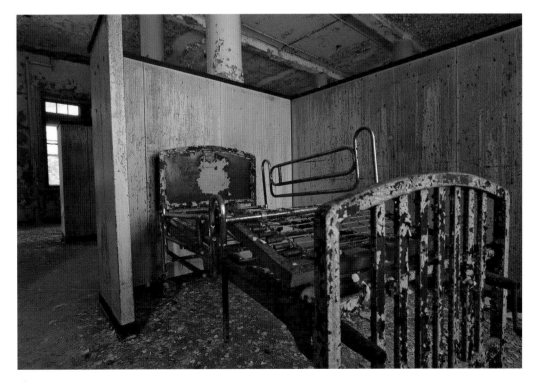

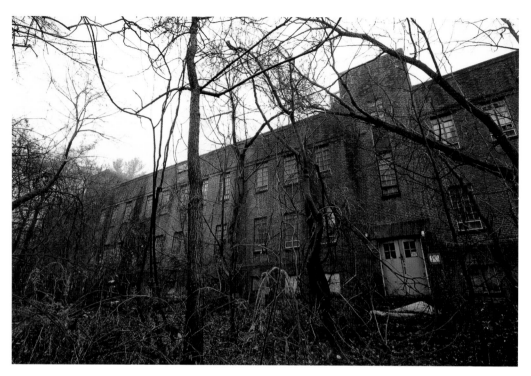

Some regions of the grounds have become thoroughly reclaimed by the forest; in this case, an entire three-story building has been assimilated by the ever-encroaching wood line.

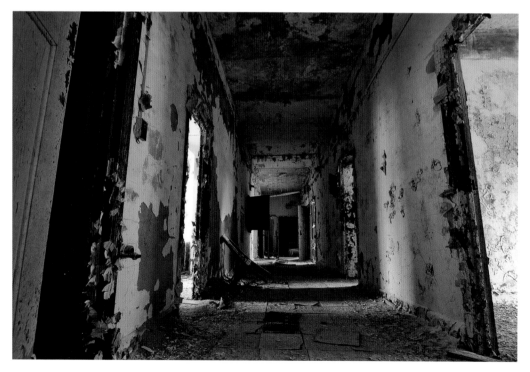

In many ways, some obvious and some subtle, the forest that has come to claim the exterior of this building is also slowly finding its way inside. Nature is constant and infinitely patient.

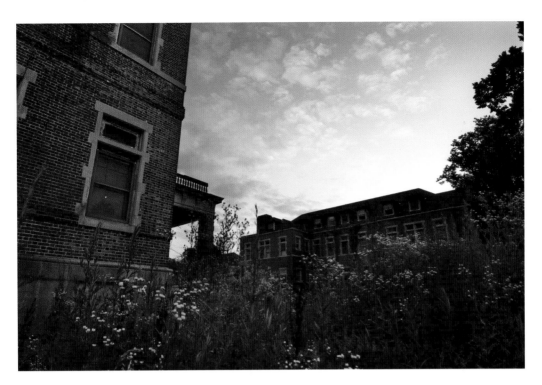

As the sun began its descent beyond the horizon, and the old Pennhurst grounds became bathed in hues of amber and red, a strange feeling of calm flowed over the grounds. It was almost as if the hospital itself was settling in for the night ahead.

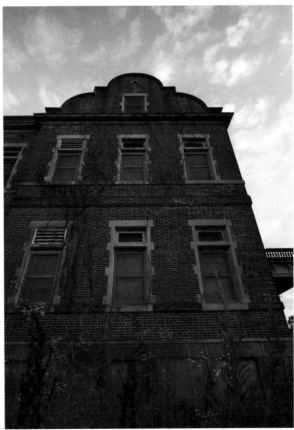

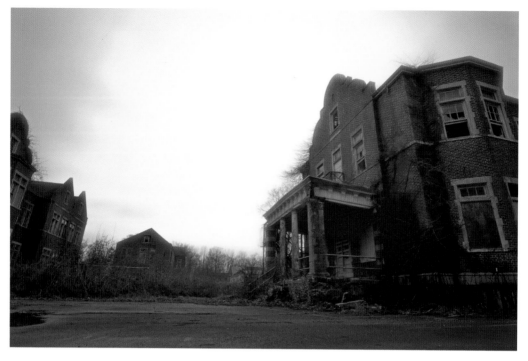

The warm-colored washes of sunset were fleeting, and it was not long until dusk and the deep blues of night crept across the grounds. The woods, which were silent during the daylight hours, were now alive with all manner of nocturnal creature, their cries and calls beckoning to one another in darkness.

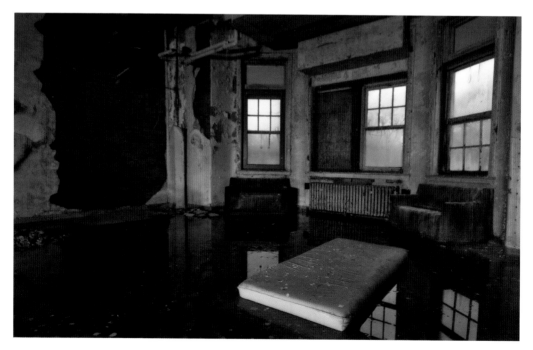

After sundown, the asylum is something completely different. The inky gloom that blots out the corridors and far corners of rooms create a space that feels many times smaller than that during the day—as if the darkness itself were taking up the space all around you.

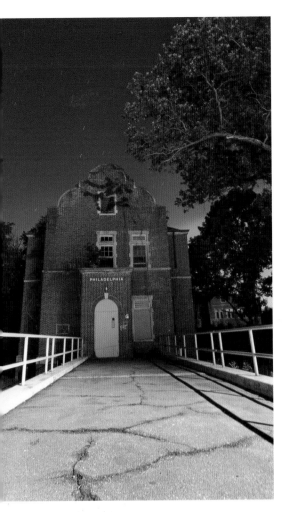
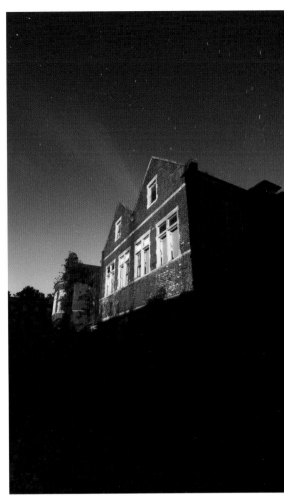

Outside in the night air, the darkness seemed far less claustrophobic, and the skies above glowed with a beautiful radiance as the purple of the night sky transitioned to an orange glow cast by the neighboring township.

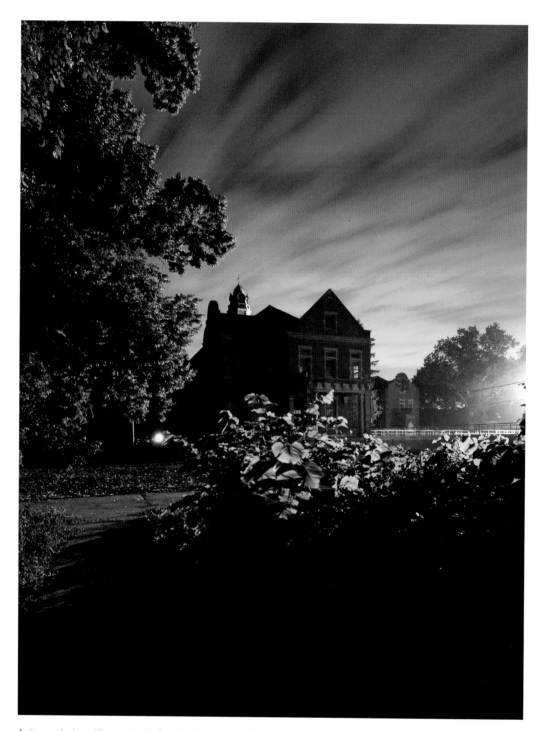

A strange juxtaposition was to be found between that celestial beauty and these storied shells on earth. Still, that is the point of all this, is it not? To see things in a new light, and by that light perhaps glean a better understanding for what it is you are gazing upon. Pennhurst is beautiful, in the same way the tragic hero of a classic story is: flawed, and eventually undone by its own failings, and for better or worse, we see our humanity in it. Pennhurst was destined to fail from its onset, and to many it now exists as a sad reminder of our wrongs. That much may be true, but does it not also serve as a poignant physical reminder of how far we have come since those times?

2

BELCHERTOWN STATE SCHOOL FOR THE FEEBLE-MINDED

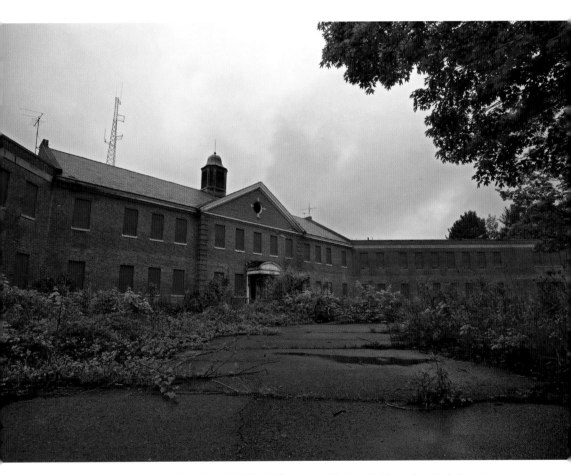

Belchertown State School for the Feeble-Minded first opened its doors in Massachusetts in the autumn of 1922. At its peak, it sprawled itself across a campus of nearly 900 acres; however, upon our visit to these grounds that fact was hardly evident. The foliage had so overtaken the long-abandoned property that one could barely lay eyes upon the next closest building, let alone gaze over any real distance.

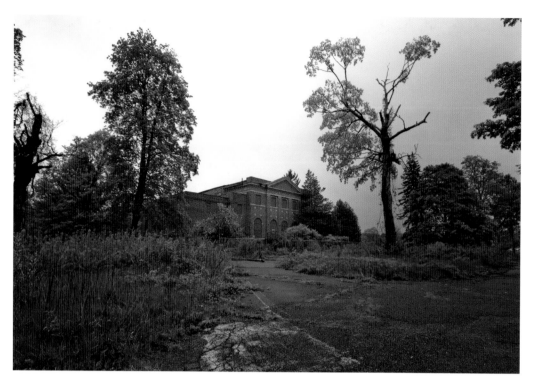

The facility operated as a cottage-style campus, with numerous independent structures dotting the landscape, each serving a particular role in the daily activity of the school. After being left abandoned in 1992, the nearby woods were quick to reclaim the lawns and open spaces between buildings, resulting in a sprawling forest punctuated with decaying husks of red brick.

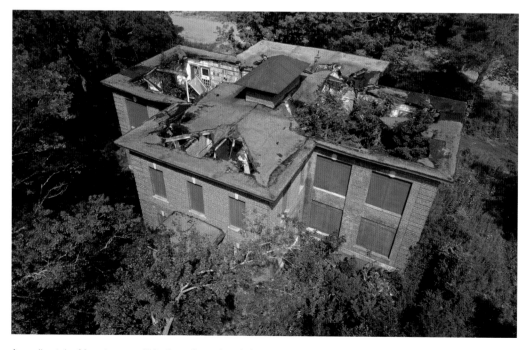

A small patch of forest grows within the collapsed roof of a ward building.

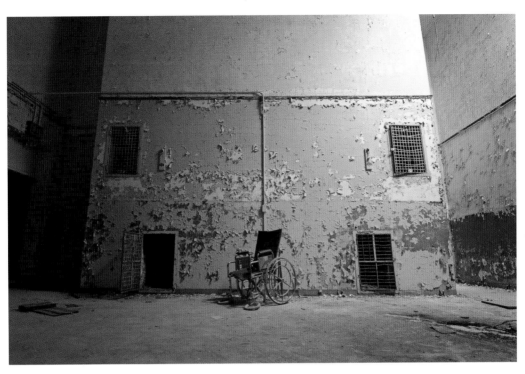

The eventual closure of Belchertown was the result of not only dwindling patient population, but a series of terrible lawsuits brought on by rampant accounts of patient neglect and abuse. Understaffing and gross overcrowding led to patients lying about in halls, moaning in distress, often injured, and covered in filth. When Francis B. Burch, the acting attorney general of Massachusetts at the time, paid a visit to the grounds, he famously referred to the school as "a hell hole."

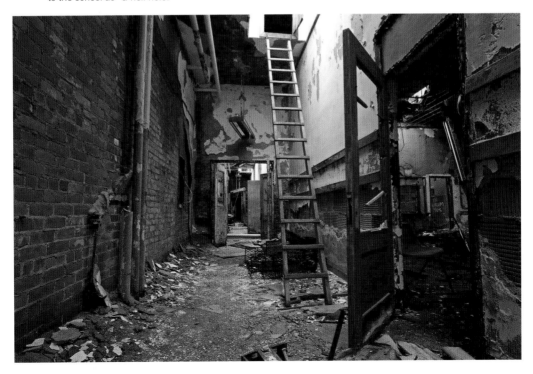

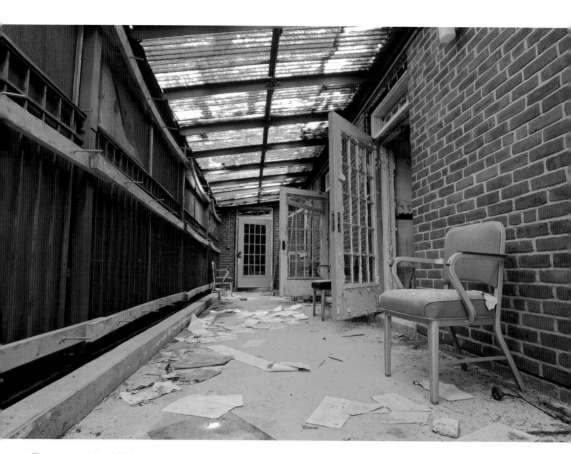

The outer porches of this therapy building were roofed in a translucent green material, which cast an eerie green glow across more than half of the upper floor of the building. The only portions not washed in the hue were the far-off corners of pitch black, where no light could reach.

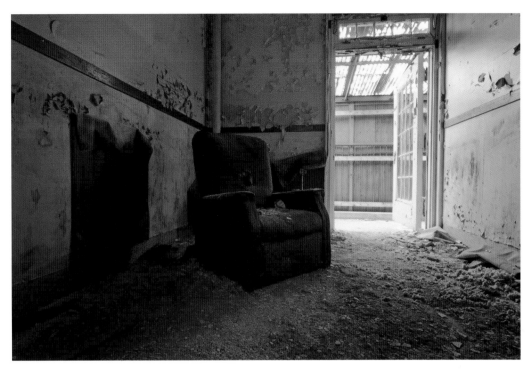

Alone in a room, an armchair slowly decomposes, bathed in a luminous green. When left behind, chairs more than most any other item seem to exude a contemplative air, as if reflecting upon what they may have seen through the years.

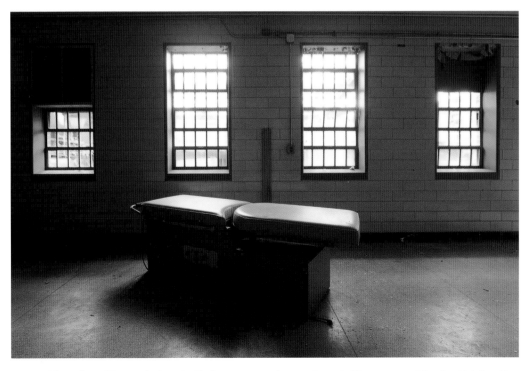

A long-disused therapy bed, washed in the same green hues as the rest of the upper-most floor in which it resides.

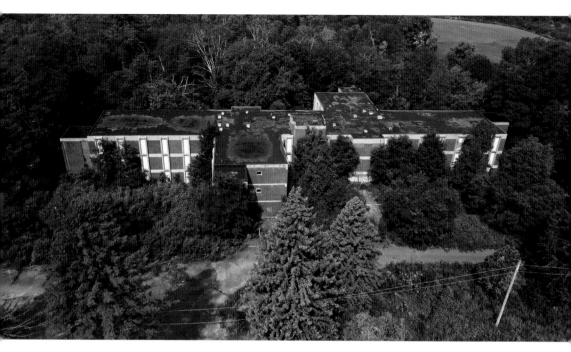

In some areas, the tips of trees stood well above the rooftop, and if you look closely, you can still make out where square patches of mowed lawn once were, replaced now by tangled underbrush and briers.

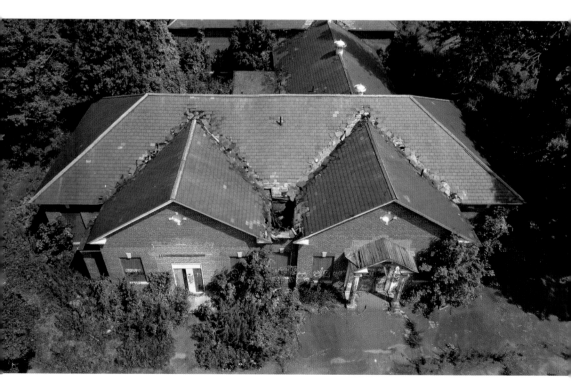

The state of weathering is far more visible from above. Here the roofing joints and seams have failed, and the slate shingles have fallen away, allowing rain and snow easy entrance to the already jeopardized building.

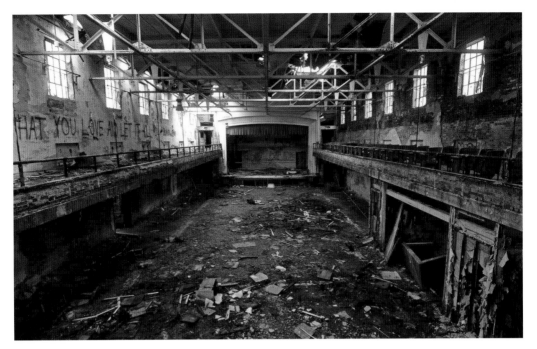

By far the most renowned building on the Belchertown grounds was the old auditorium. It was also one of the most severely decayed structures, making for a haunting visual when one considers just how many once gathered here during the heyday of the school.

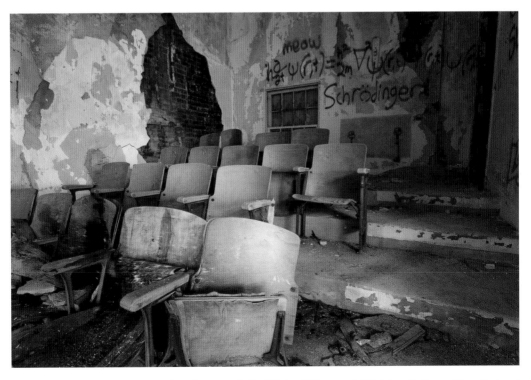

In the absence of crowds and applause, one instead finds wild ferns rooted in fallen plaster, and the chirping of birds that have come to nest in the exposed roof supports.

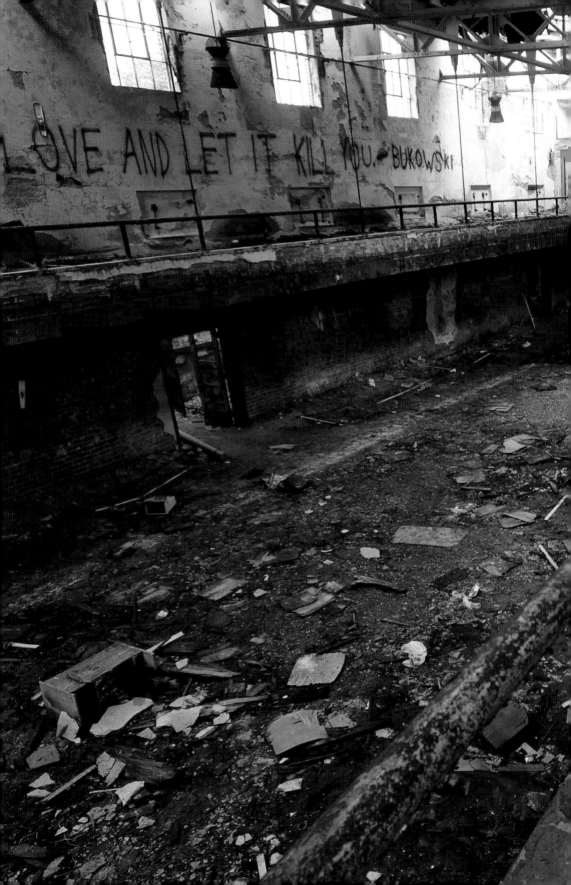

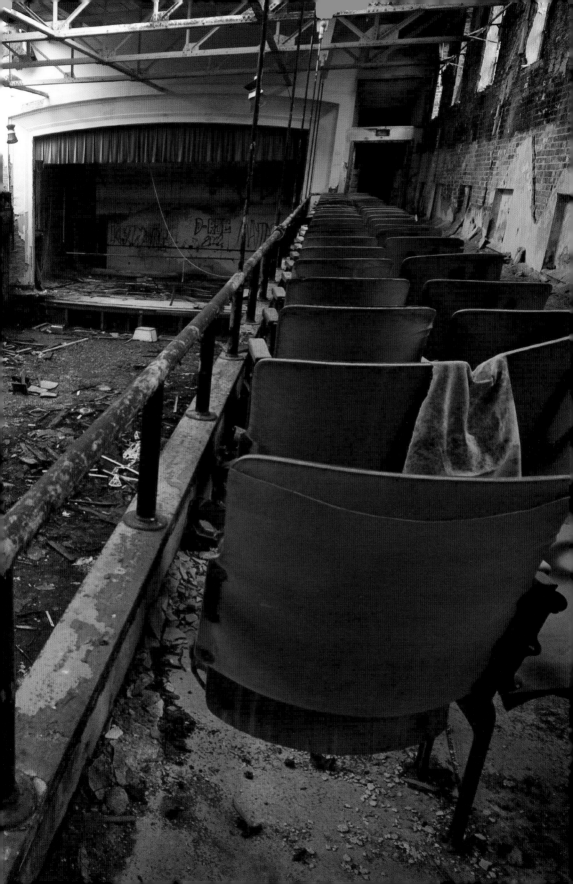

Previous page: The upper-level seating of the old auditorium had existed for years with very little roof remaining over it, and through this a surreal mingling of nature and manmade had occurred. Though, when one truly thinks upon it, the natural and manmade worlds are not all that different. In the end, it all turns to dirt, and as of 2015, as much could be said for the entirety of this auditorium—having been razed to make way for redevelopment of the grounds.

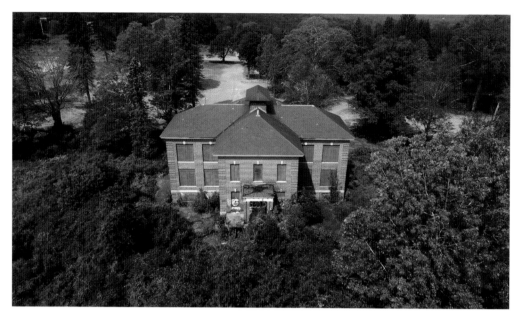

By this point in time, demolition had claimed most of the central campus, but there remained many holdouts in the tree line, awaiting their fate.

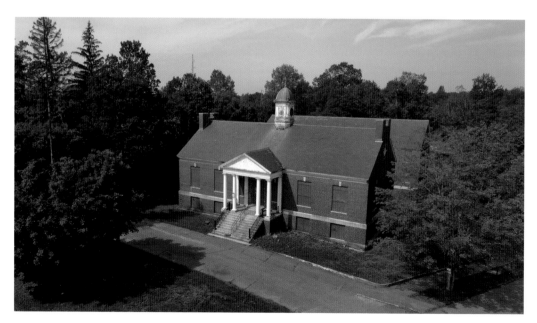

The old administration building still greets visitors at the entrance to the grounds. Through the years, its clock tower has come to be a trademark of the old Belchertown school grounds, and perhaps it will remain so. This building is slated to be preserved and adaptively reused into the future development of the property.

3

NORWICH STATE HOSPITAL FOR THE INSANE

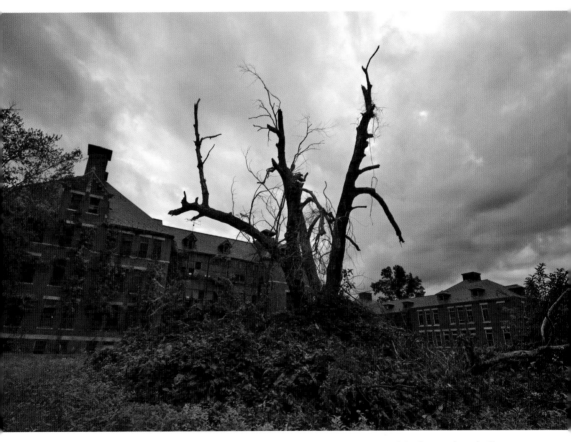

Norwich State Hospital opened its doors in the towns of Preston and Norwich, Connecticut, in the autumn of 1904. At the time, the initial patient count at the new facility was under 100. However, not unlike numerous institutions of its day, the patient population at the hospital grew exponentially. By 1930, Norwich had sprawled itself out from a single hospital center to a campus of over twenty buildings.

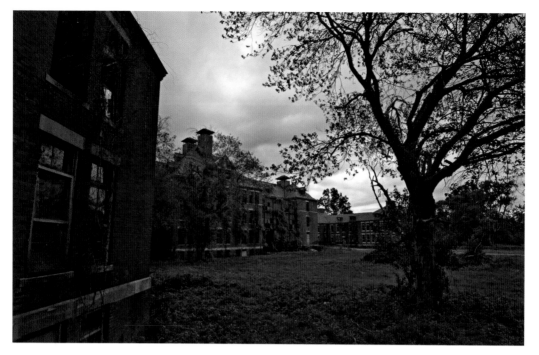

Every so often, one may find themselves in a place where it seems that the environment itself has been deeply affected by the history that it bore. Even the trees here loomed over the campus in an otherworldly way—secretive, gnarled things that seemed to whisper among themselves at the very edge of hearing.

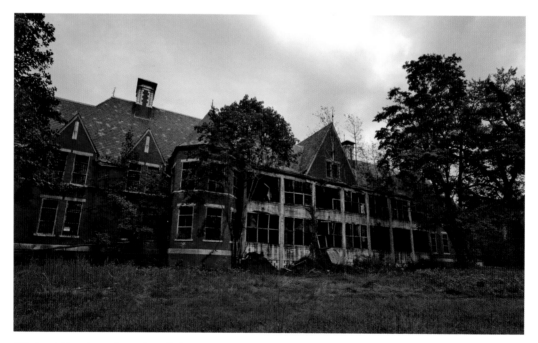

Pitted metal bars framed countless windows that overlooked the decayed grounds of the long-abandoned asylum. Upon our visit, this old campus was little more than a gathering of sad and rotten buildings, but if one were to have peered out those same windows some seventy years earlier, they would have seen a massive city operating unto itself, with a populace in the thousands.

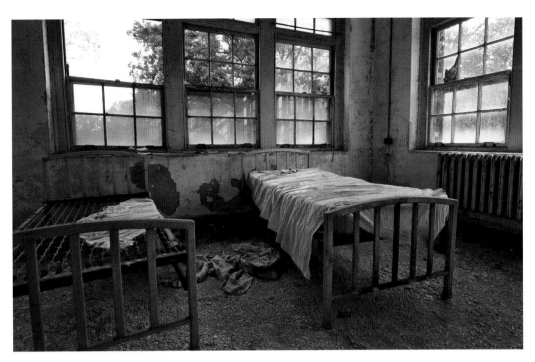

A ward of beds rot away. Even after decades of disuse, discolored linens remained on several of the beds.

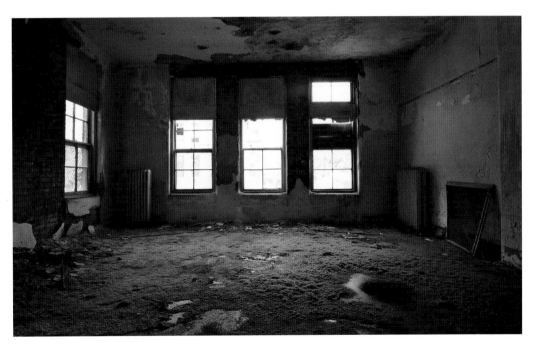

Years of leaky roofing had allowed for a thick layer of moss to cover many floors of the old asylum. It is in these ephemeral instances wherein nature and manmade slowly merge that one feels a powerful mixture of humbling awe.

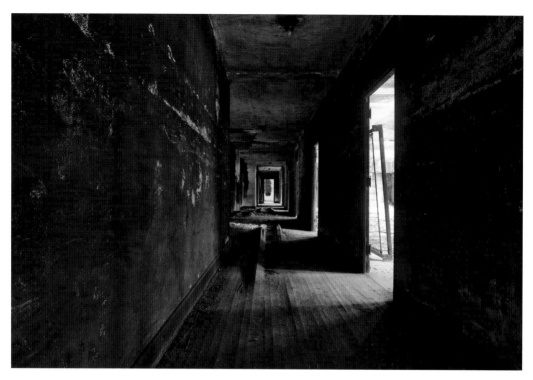

Little remained here, save for shadows—an ever-present substance that had made a home in every corner and corridor of the campus.

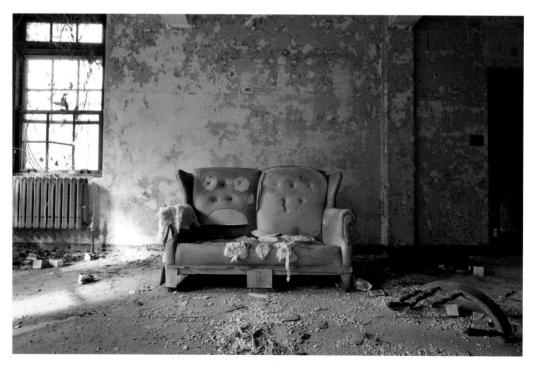

When left behind, simple everyday objects—in this case a decrepit couch—become captivating focal points. Perhaps it is that they now sit alone in places that had once been so full of life.

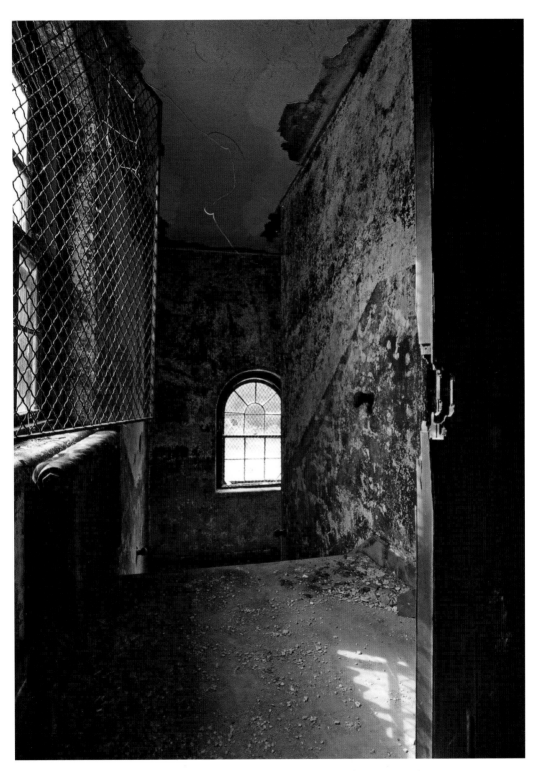

As the years went on, the population of the campus eventually began to decrease due to modern psychiatric medications, and the growing taboo that the country was beginning to feel toward large state institutions. During this time, Norwich began constructing new modern buildings on a plot of property next to where the old hospital center stood.

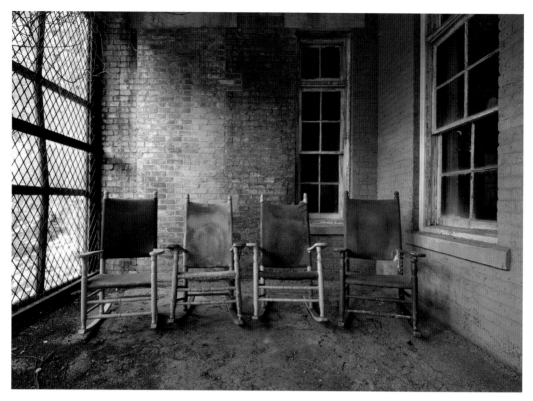

Every time a new building on the modern hospital campus was constructed and opened, a building from the old hospital campus was closed down.

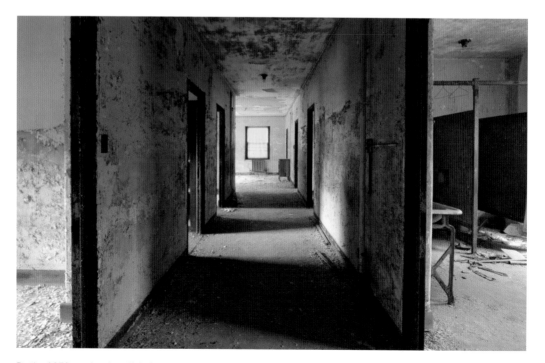

By the 1970s, only a handful of the original asylum buildings were in active use.

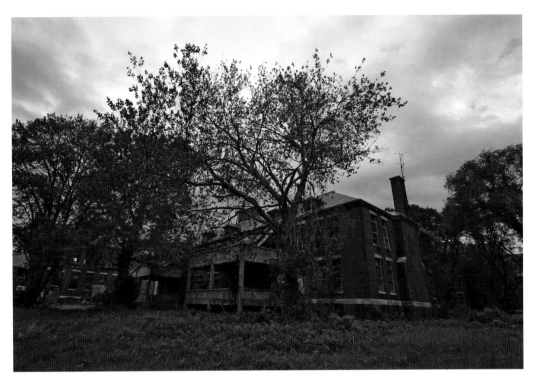

When the Norwich State Hospital finally shuttered in 1996, only two of the original campus buildings were still in use, with the remainders of the old campus already falling into disrepair.

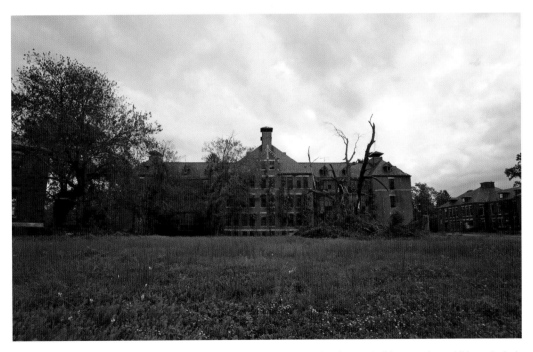

It was the beautiful architecture of the original asylum campus that drew us to this property, and it is exclusively these buildings that we documented during our visit. Though the new campus surely has its own stories to tell, those modern buildings have not a shadow of the character that was found on the grounds of the old hospital.

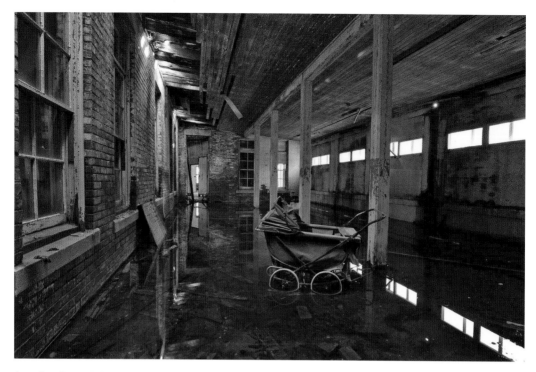

A stroller sits partially submerged on the flooded floor of a badly decayed ward—a bizarre scene that seems somehow at home on the Norwich grounds.

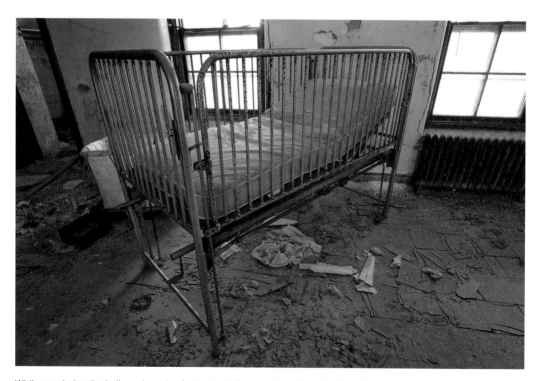

While wandering the halls and wards of state institutions such as Norwich, it can be easy to begin to forget just who the people were who called these chambers home, but the hospital is quick with reminders.

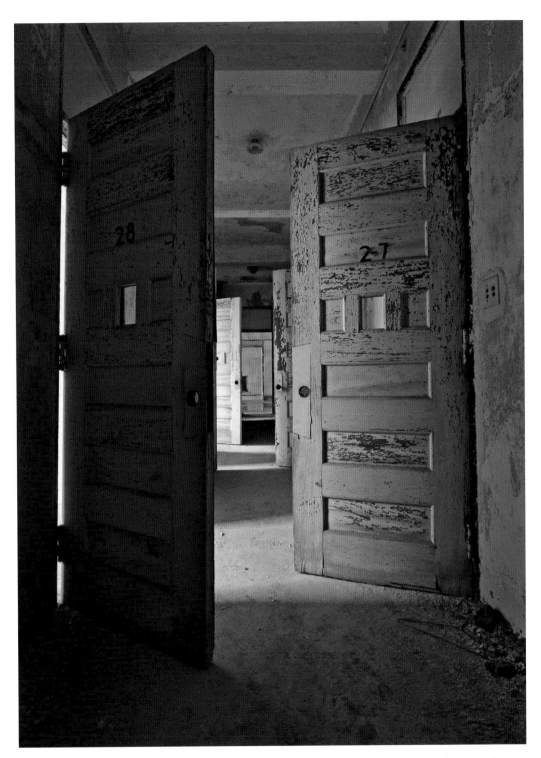

The most overwhelming thing about spending any length of time in an abandoned institution is not what one would initially expect. The stories of abuse and neglect are deeply upsetting, and the need to be on constant guard not only from the jeopardized building structure, but from wild animals can make one weary. However, what weighs most heavily upon your mind while walking these halls is the utter silence all around you. It is inescapable.

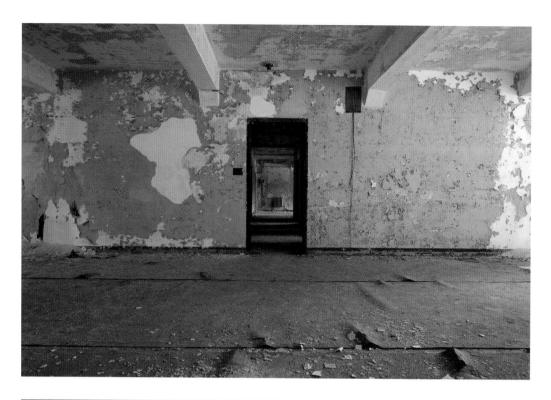

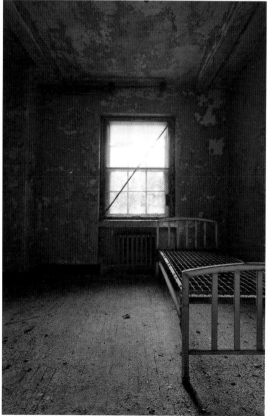

Above: A doorway leads away from a large dayroom to a crooked corridor of black.

Left: A patient bedroom perpetually shadowed, mutely saying much.

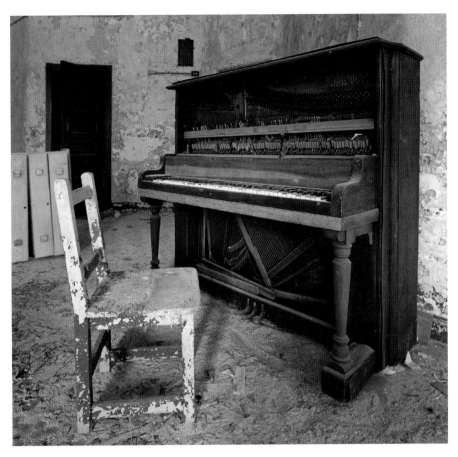

At least one piano can be found in nearly every abandoned mental institution, often left behind when institutions close down simply because of the difficulty of removing it. When abandoned along with the buildings, they become significant relics, in no small part due to the role that music played in patient therapy, as well as the daily life on a ward. In just a few years' time, the pianos become ruined by humidity and temperature, reduced to sad reminders of times gone by.

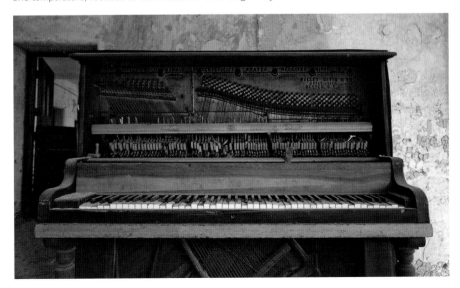

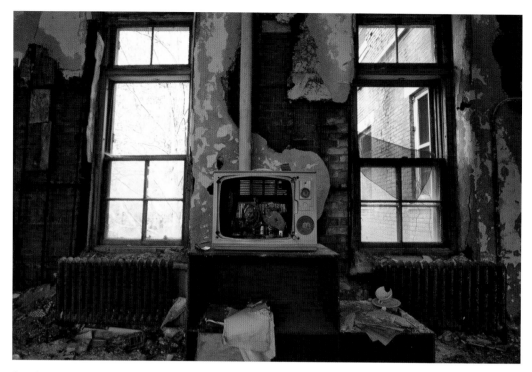

Over time, radio and television became utilized less to entertain patients and more to distract and pacify, especially during times of overcrowding and understaffing, which came to plague institutions such as Norwich.

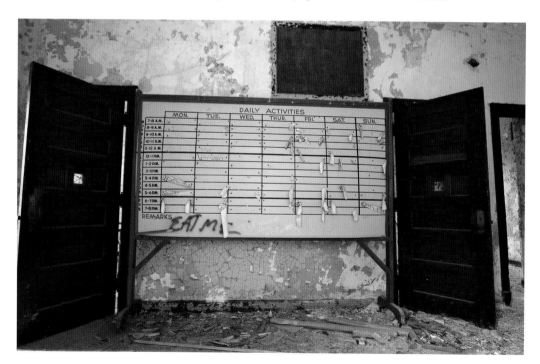

A patient activity board stands against a wall in a common room. Most of the activity notes have long been lost to the ages, but some remain, such as "supper" from 5–6 p.m. and "evening news" from 6–7 p.m. Faint glimpses at the daily lives of those who were here before us.

Though surely a trying environment at many times for both patients and staff, it was also clear from items left behind that the hospital did attempt to do right by those they were tasked with caring for. Here we find a large wooden box, decorated to look as a brick chimney topped with snow. On the side reads "Christmas Gifts for patients. Norwich Hospital." The old campus, though troubled, surely must have been a sight during the holiday season.

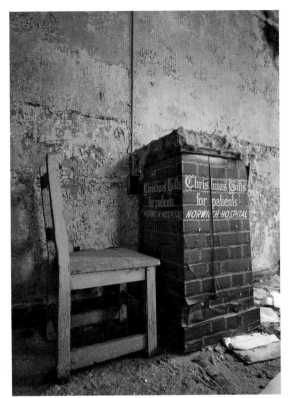

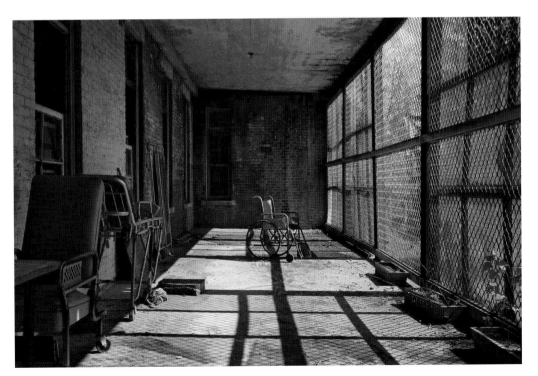

A wheelchair looks outward from the second floor of an enclosed porch. A view from which it may well have watched the rise and fall of the hospital, now overgrown and mostly forgotten.

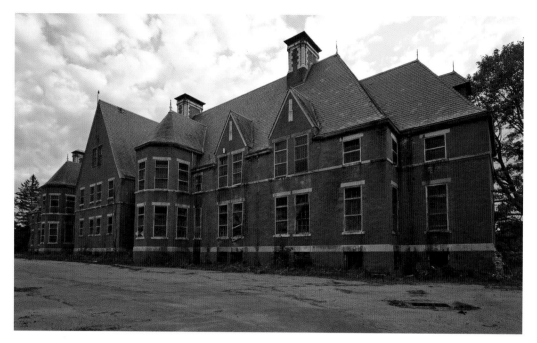

The old Norwich grounds were a beautiful collection of red brick cottage-style buildings, spaced across a campus that had come to take on an increasingly surreal atmosphere the longer it sat disused. Today, though, if you visit the grounds you will find little more than a grassy field where the historic asylum once stood. Demolition began on the property in 2011, and over several years, nearly every building on the old campus was razed with the exception of the administration, which is currently mothballed to be utilized in the future development of the grounds, whatever and whenever they may be.

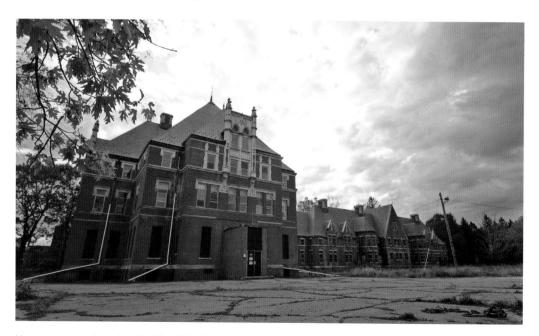

Here you can see the admin building (left side of frame) with new windows and a sealed lower floor. Hopefully, when the site is eventually redeveloped, the preserved admin building may serve to help tell the story of what once stood on these grounds.

4

LETCHWORTH VILLAGE

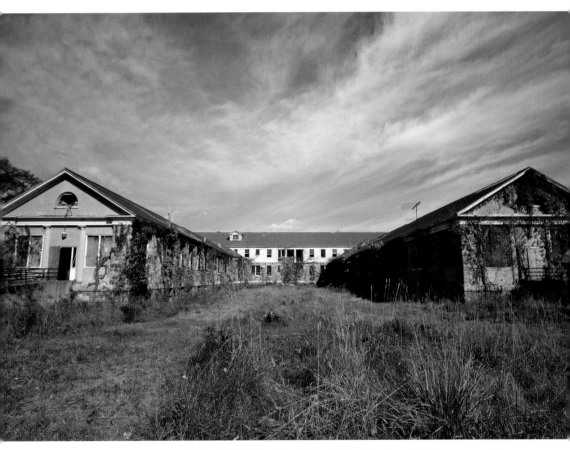

In 1909, on a rolling parcel of land in Rockland County, New York, a brand new facility was opened for the aid and housing of—as the literature declares—the "feeble minded and epileptics" of that state. This new facility was called Letchworth Village, named for William Pryor Letchworth, a noted humanitarian of the time and a man who was instrumental in its creation.

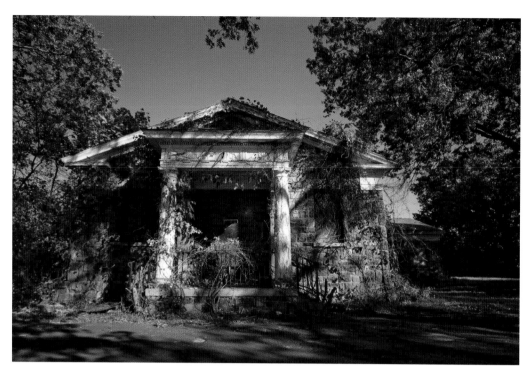

In order to avoid creating an institutional environment for the patients, the grounds of Letchworth Village were arranged much like a college campus, with a multitude of structures dotting the landscape. The buildings were relatively small, typically not exceeding two stories in height, and were inspired by the aesthetics of Greek architecture. Walls of hand-cut stone punctuated by arched windows and column-girded doorways can still be found at every turn, though today much is concealed by twisting ivy.

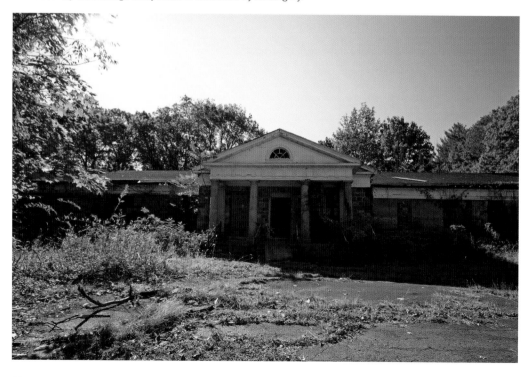

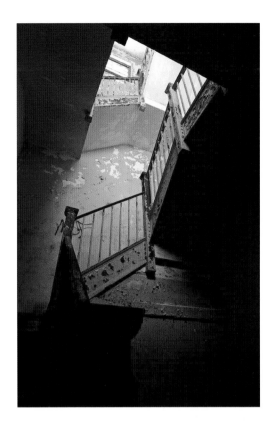

A staircase leads skyward from the basement, towards daylight and the floors above.

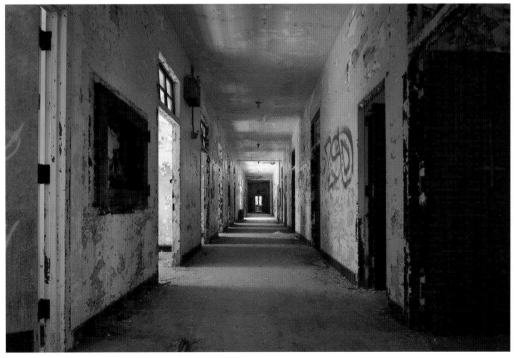

The doors along this upper corridor are slammed open and shut all day by the wind, which continuously rushes through many broken and missing window panes.

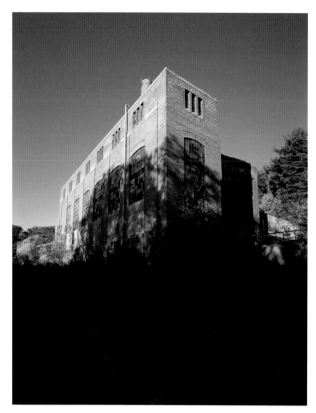

Short walks across grassy lawns separated the buildings and the greater campus, which housed its own power plant, farmland, waste disposal, and water supply. The power plant still stands today, lost beyond a thick wall of trees.

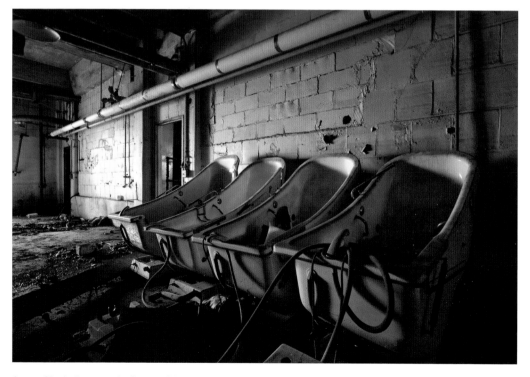

A row of hydrotherapy tubs line a wall in the basement of the old power plant.

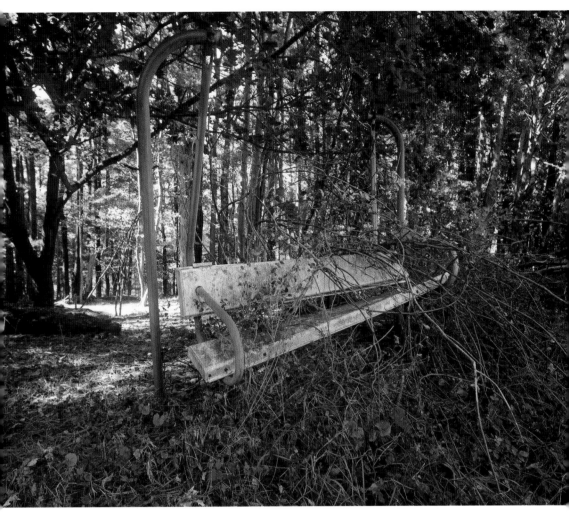

A darker part of Letchworth's history that is of great note is that, beyond serving as an asylum, the facility was also utilized for medical research. Most famously, it served in the development of the polio vaccines used in the Congo by Dr. Hilary Koprowski. To those ends, twenty "mentally deficient" inhabitants of Letchworth Village served Koprowski as the first human test subjects to be injected with the vaccine.

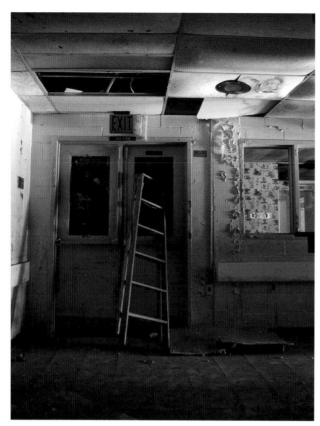

Whereas we mentioned that the original campus buildings were designed to create as little of an institutional air as possible, the later structures that were built paid little heed to that mindset. Stacked cinder block replaced hand-cut stone, and plasterwork was replaced by sheetrock and drop-ceiling. These buildings also paid less attention to accessible daylight, and for that they were much darker within.

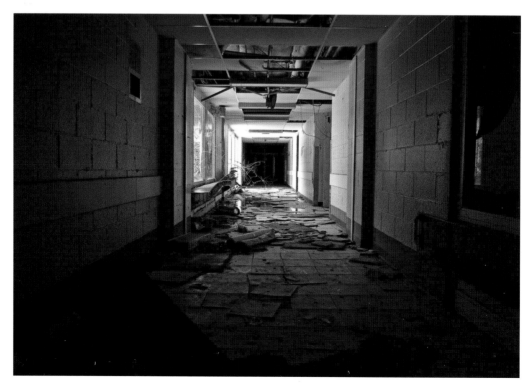

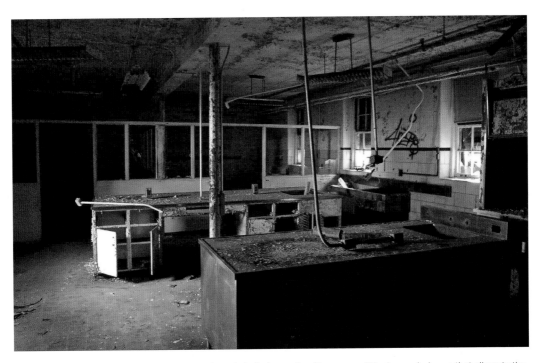

Light creeps in through the seams in boarded windows, dispelling some of the heavy darkness that clings to the basement laboratory and autopsy room.

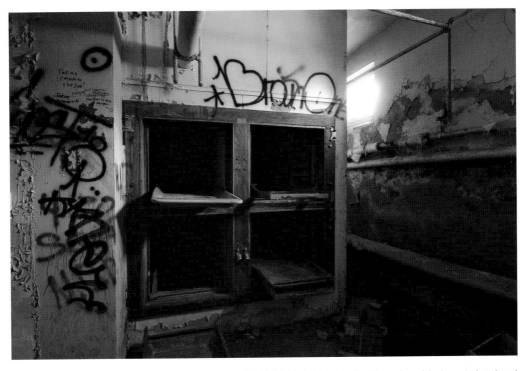

A four-drawer morgue resides in the basement of Kirkbride Hall at Letchworth Village. One of the largest abandoned structures on the campus, it was utilized for a wide variety of purposes throughout its service—lastly as an administration building.

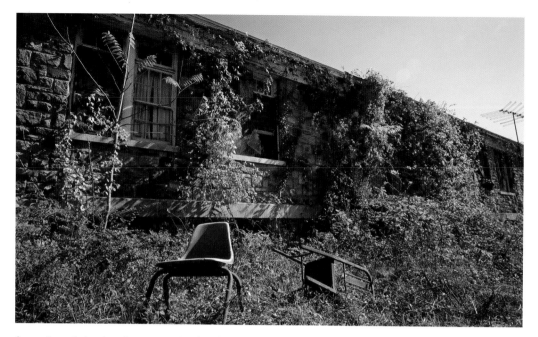

As was the unfortunate pattern among state hospitals, the gradual decline of Letchworth began with overcrowding. Along with many United States psychiatric hospitals, the 1950s through the 1970s saw a huge increase in patient population, well beyond those for which the facility was designed. Additionally, a documentary titled *The Last Disgrace* was made, focusing on the sad condition of these hospitals by the then-local reporter Geraldo Rivera, who brought the situation at Letchworth (and similarly run institutions nationwide) to the public eye.

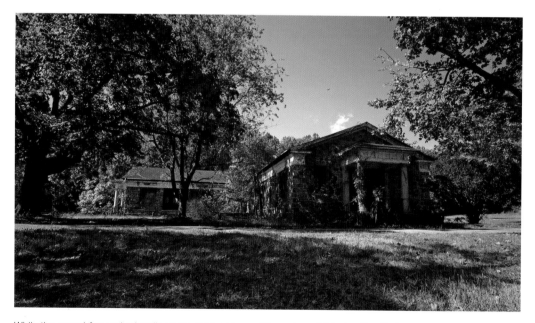

While the exposé focused primarily on the deplorable conditions at a neighboring New York state asylum called Willowbrook, Letchworth was featured in a substantial segment of the final work. When ABC aired the piece, it resulted in a massive public outcry for the betterment of patient care. This trend, coupled with a shift toward mental care on a smaller scale, resulted in the slow redistribution of Letchworth's patients to other locations. In 1997, the last of the residents were relocated, and the village's long-running independent utility grid was shut down forever.

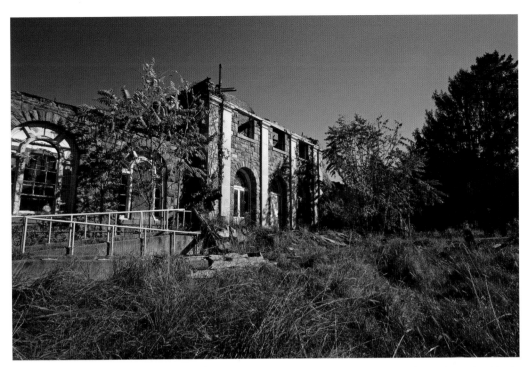

A fire decimated this amusement hall building in the summer of 2010. Today, it stands as a burned-out husk, and fallen columns and glassless arched windows hint at the grandeur that once was.

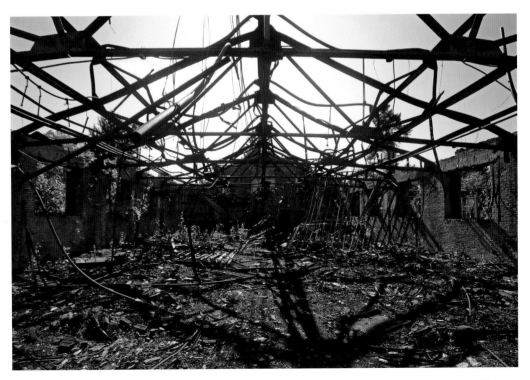

Within, plant life has begun to reclaim the scorched earth, helped along by sunlight and rainwater, which now cascade through the destroyed roof.

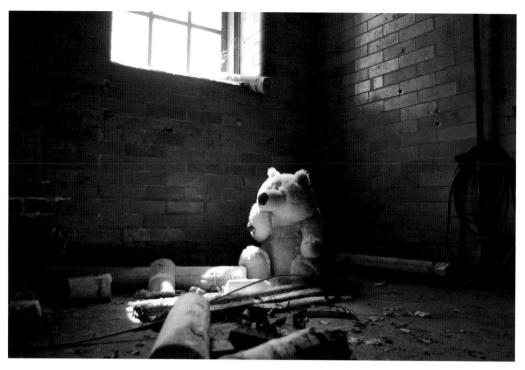

An orphaned stuffed bear remains behind on the floor of a storage room.

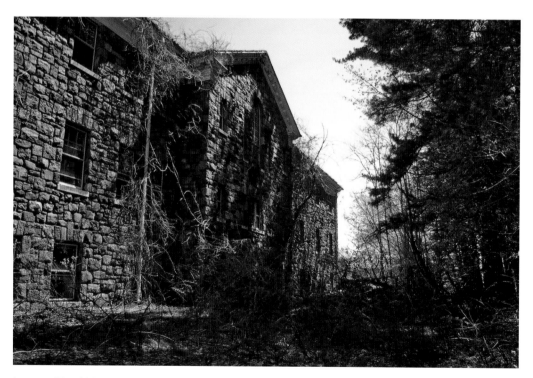

In researching this location, we have found that even a passing mention of its name is bound to bring out ghost stories. Abandoned places, especially asylums, often serve as the spark for countless tales of the paranormal tales, and Letchworth seems to be a particular favorite.

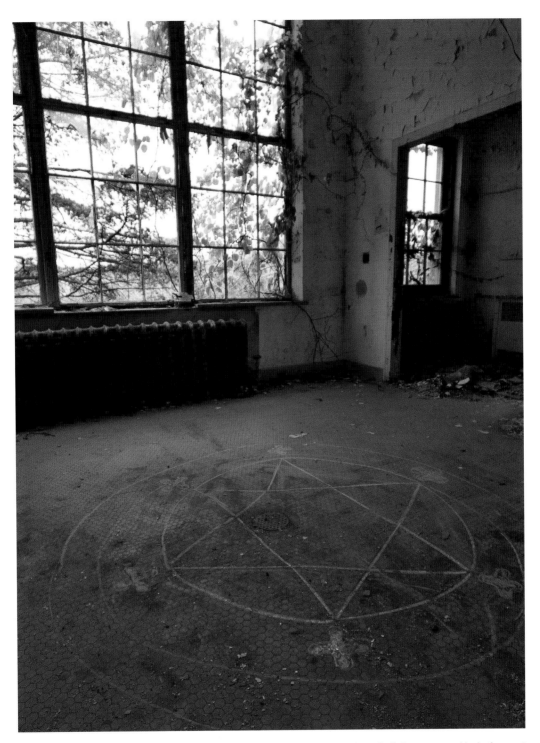

Unfortunately, this interest seems to come with a lot of baggage attached, particularly an apparent lack of respect for the grounds—respect for the history, which runs through the walls of places such as Letchworth Village, and respect for people who lived and died here. Perhaps the most heartbreaking for us, though, is to see empathy replaced by exploitation, particularly of the people who endured lives of unimaginable isolation and pain here, tormented by the demons of their own minds that the medicine of the era was helpless to cure.

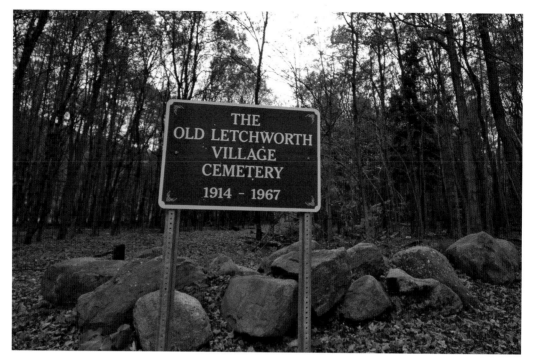

Many of those who lived and died at Letchworth Village remain here to this day. While some may go hunting for apparitions in the shadowy corridors and peeling wards, if you truly wish to visit with them, they rest eternal just a short drive from the campus proper, off Call Hollow Road.

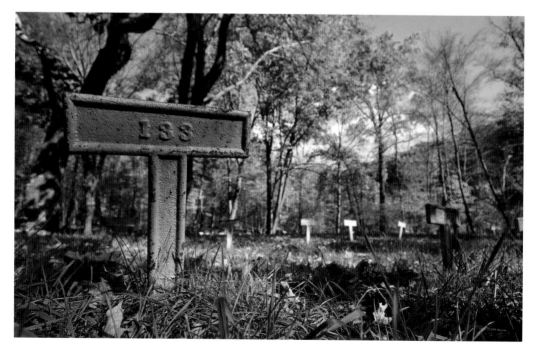

As was customary practice, many residents at not just Letchworth Village, but nationwide, were given numbers as identifiers in place of names. Sadly, these numbers followed them to their final resting place, with a simple numerical plaque signifying who lays beneath.

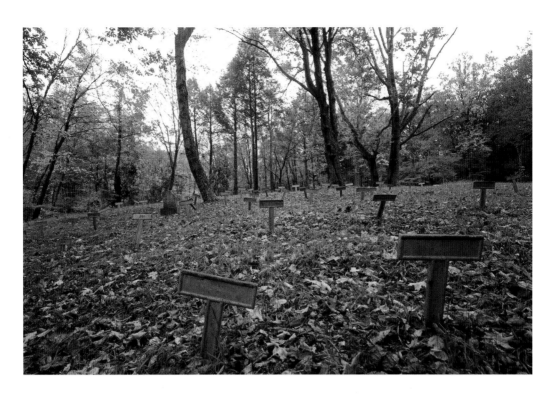

Above: If you seek to better understand what Letchworth Village was and who called it home, sit for some time among the numbered dead.

Right: Correcting Wrongs: Years ago, a small monument was installed at the entry to the cemetery, upon it reads the names of those interred here.

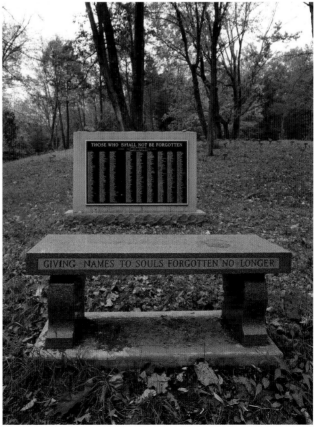

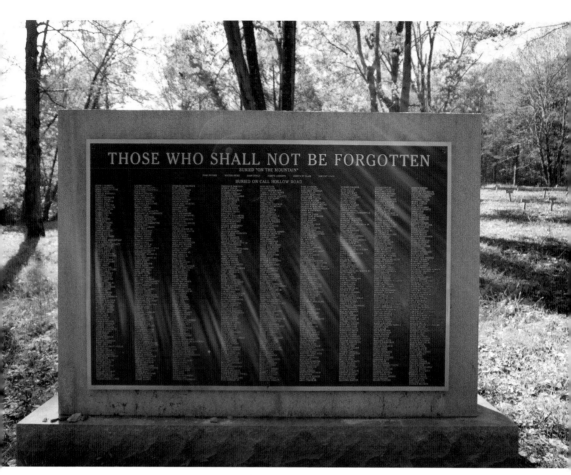

Though the cemetery is barely visited today, and the path to reach it winds through rocks, downed trees, and mud, it is forever a resting place to some 900 souls. They now rest with some dignity restored.

5

THE "PSYCHOPATHIC BUILDING"

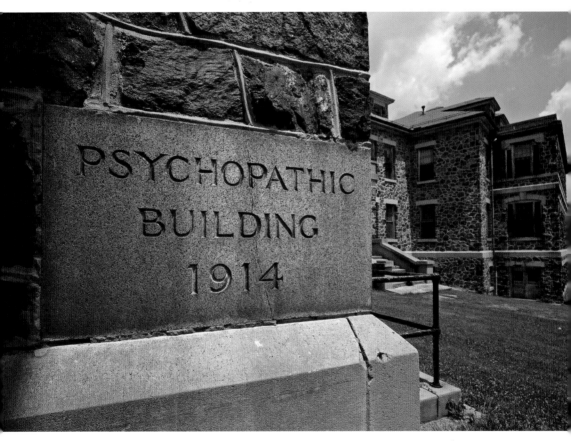

In the heart of a partially-active Spring Grove Hospital Center in Maryland, surrounded by neatly mowed lawns and busy roadways, sits the neglected remains of one of its founders and originators. A boldly cut cornerstone on the face of the weathered building proclaims this to be the "Psychopathic Building." Below that, in the same pronounced print, one finds its date of birth: 1914.

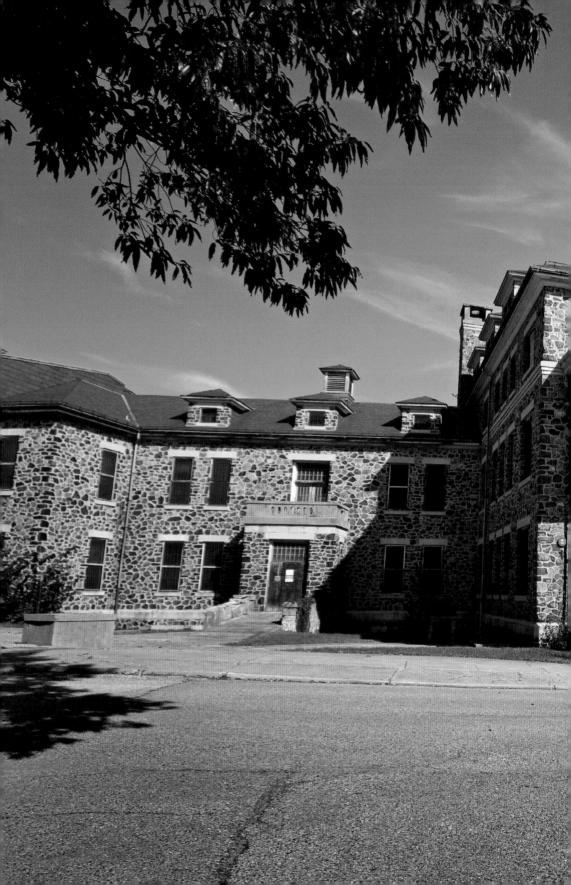

Like many buildings hailing from this era of American architecture, the "Psychopathic Building" radiates character. You simply do not see these kinds of buildings anymore. Obviously, the primary reason for this is due to expense, but we also must wonder if perhaps any artisans even remain in the modern day who could craft such an edifice. High walls of stone frame a pillared entrance akin to the kind one may see at a grand estate. Outstretched to the left and right lie the wards. All of it is beautiful, and also sadly forgotten, even in the midst of a busy campus.

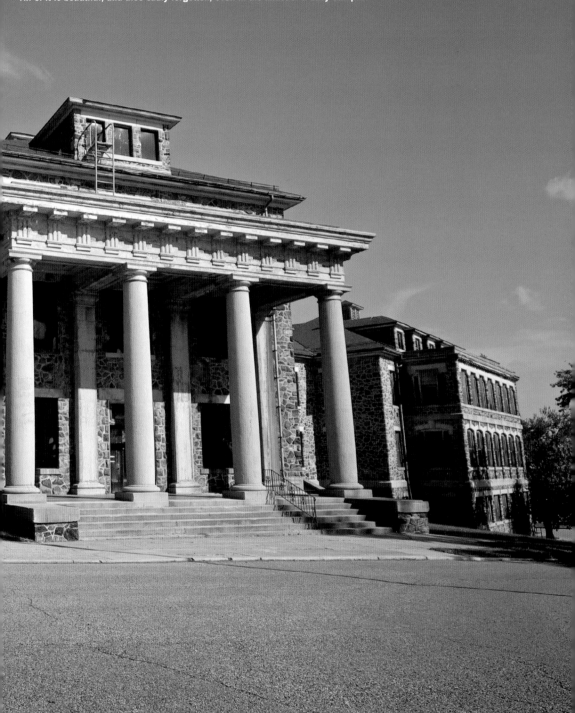

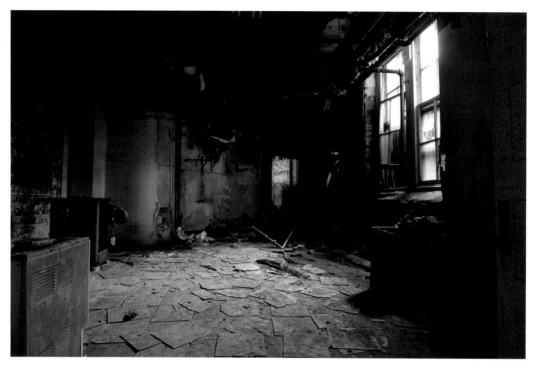

It was only 10 a.m. and the day had already reached 100 degrees, and as we walked across the sticky sun-softened pavement toward the building, we braced ourselves for what was sure to be an exceptionally warm welcome inside. We were correct. The stone walls, sealed windows, and dark roof of the asylum combined to create what was, in essence, a giant sun-oven. A near-solid wall of stagnant, humid air embraced us within moments of entering the massive building and never let go.

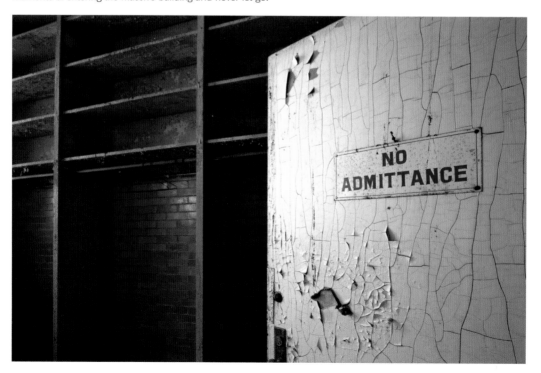

This lone wheelchair left in the basement was one of the first sights we saw upon entering. As we set up to take this photo, a kitten appeared, perched, and stared in from right outside the ground-floor window. We approached to get a better look, but the kitten quickly leapt from its perch and darted out of sight, likely rejoining the many unseen felines that we eventually learned called this place home.

All through the day, we continuously noted twisting paw-print trails leading down almost every hallway and corridor in the old hospital, clear of dust and debris from heavy use by the cat residents. Though we never saw another cat during our three hours inside, you could not shake the feeling that they were watching us from some dark corner or long shadow.

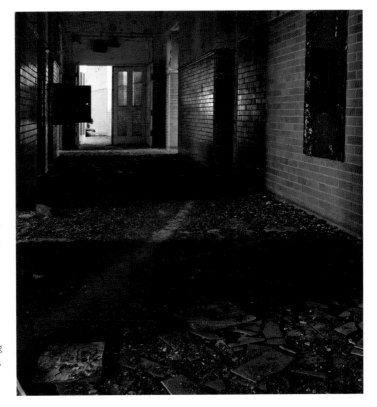

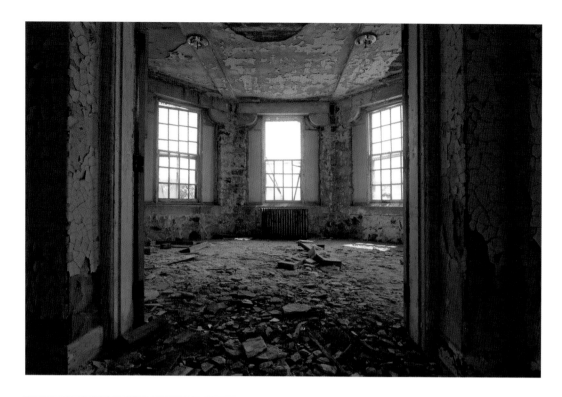

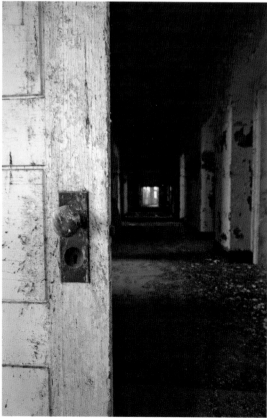

Above: A former dayroom crumbles away. Long ago, this is where patients would congregate to talk among themselves or partake in activities.

Left: For as bright as the dayrooms and bedrooms had been, the corridors and chambers between were swallowed in pitch.

Right: Unlike many of the abandoned hospital campuses we have visited, which quickly become popular hangouts for curiosity seekers or photography fodder for people such as ourselves, this building seemed to have an almost complete lack of human presence. The only visitor who frequented these halls was time.

Below: Nearly every state-run institution operated as a complete entity, separate from the greater world around it. The most obvious elements of this independence were the independent power grid, police force, and postal code, but there were also countless intimate ways, such as private patient gardens, sporting fields, and even beauty salons.

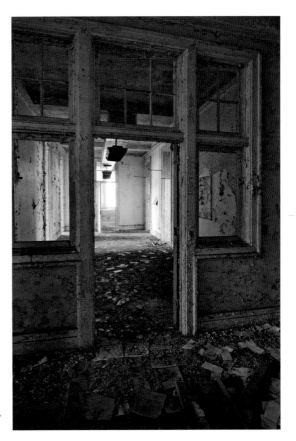

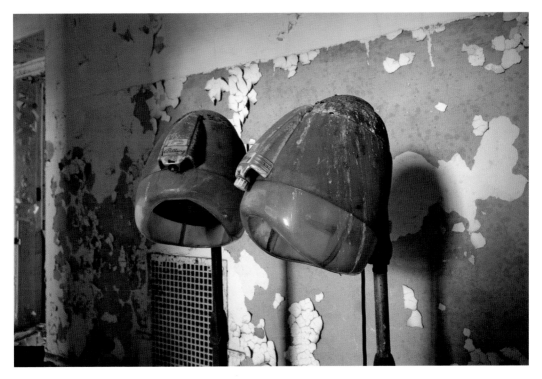

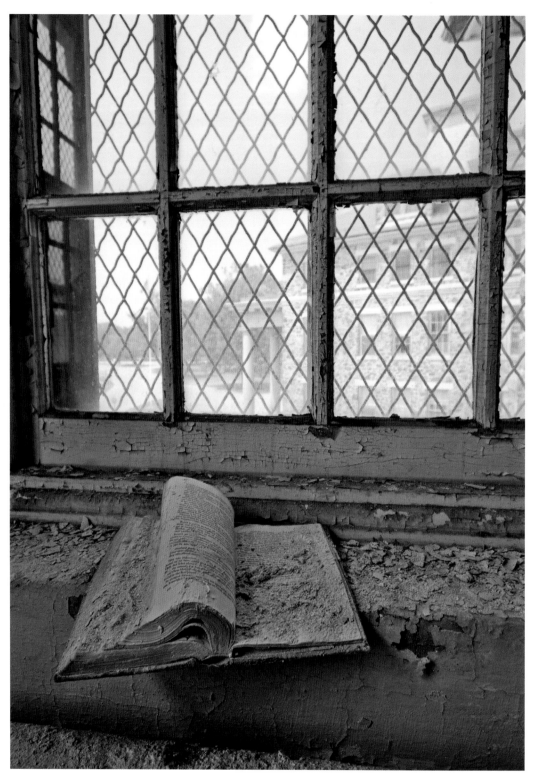

A book rests upon a ledge, perpetually half-read. The pages and binding had come to be incredibly rigid, taking on a nearly stone-like quality.

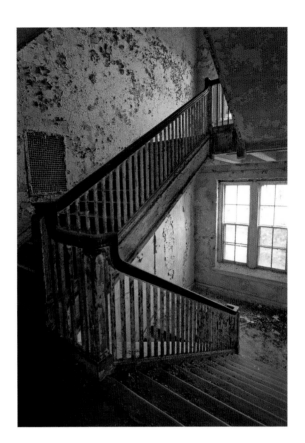

With every floor we ascended, the heat increased. The higher floors were almost unbearable to spend any length of time within. Every step taken kicked up a cloud fine dust and debris, which stuck fast to sweat-covered skin, leaving us coated in a film of grit, which did not ease our already intense discomfort.

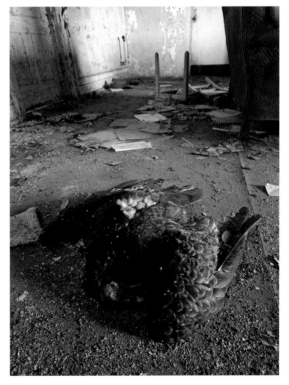

A victim of the heat. We have saved a fair share of trapped birds in sealed buildings, but we do not always arrive in time to save them all, this was sadly one of those times.

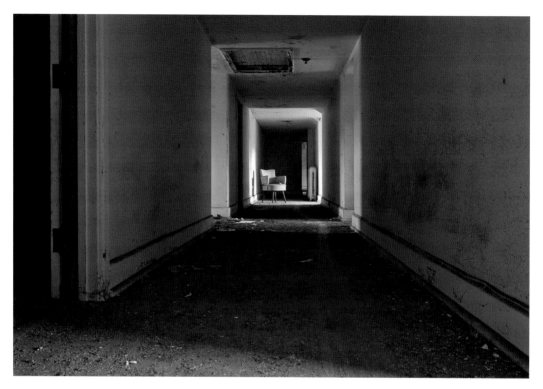

The uppermost floor of the hospital was of a different use than the wards below, set up more along the lines of apartment living than hospital residency. Being built into the inner roof of the building, there were smaller rooms, with lower, angled ceilings. This was also by far the hottest area in the whole of the hospital building.

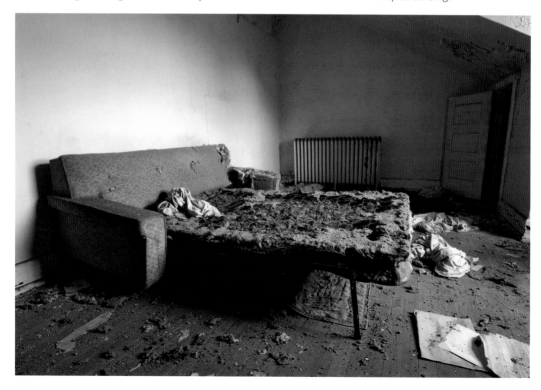

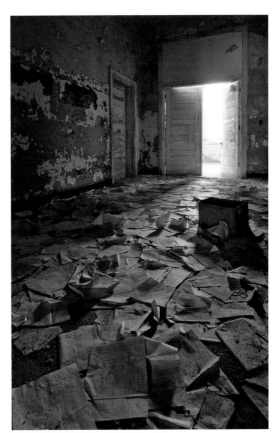

Right: A hallway strewn with paperwork, in this case mostly payment receipts for various services at the hospital.

Below: Even more paperwork, this time stored away in cardboard boxes and seemingly forgotten. Many of the storage boxes were toppled, torn, and collapsing from the years of humidity.

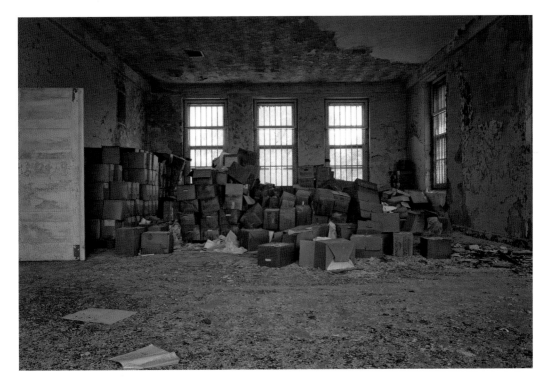

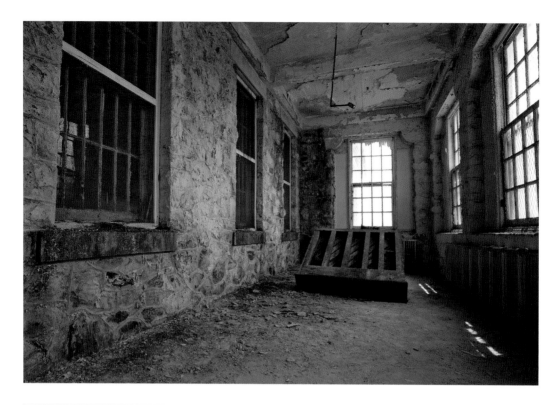

Above: A fallen stand-up piano lays broken on the floor of one of the "sun parlors," a long and narrow common room with plentiful windows specifically built to allow patients the therapeutic qualities of daylight.

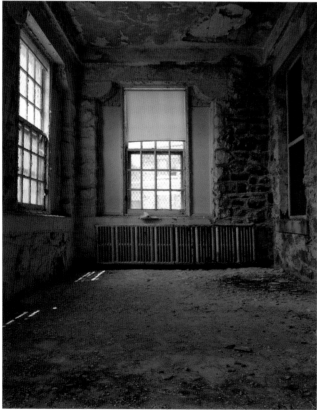

Left: The sun parlor's name belies its current state: that of an eerie and perpetually-shadowed chamber.

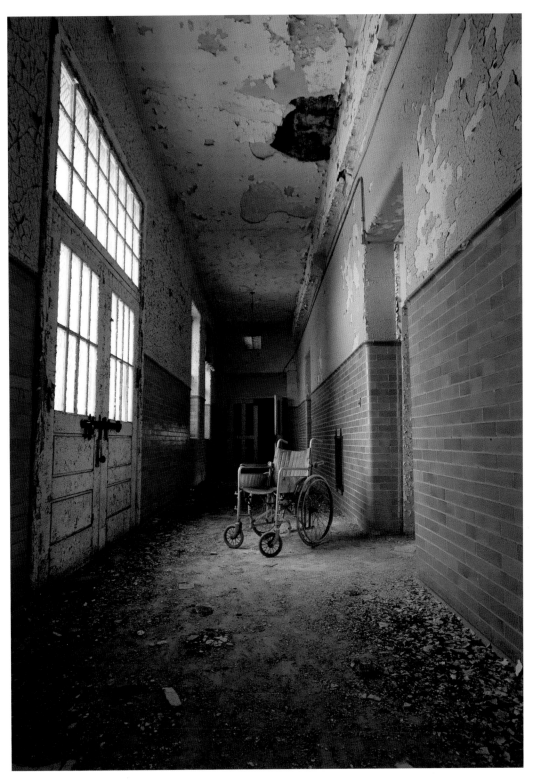

We are not alone as we trek these hospital halls. We walk these paths and halls, which countless others have walked: those who came before and those who will come after.

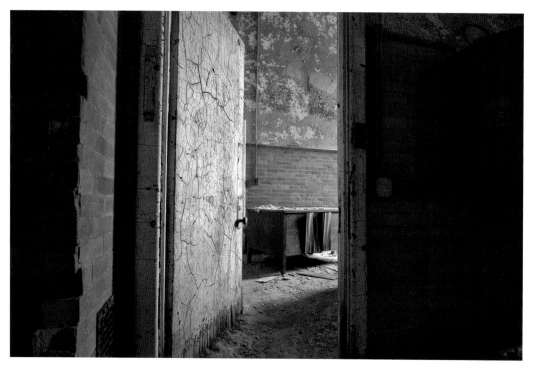

As we made our way back down and through the hospital, we came upon a severely decomposing office on the ground floor. It was an unassuming room, and sat alone at the end of a hall behind a shattered wooden door.

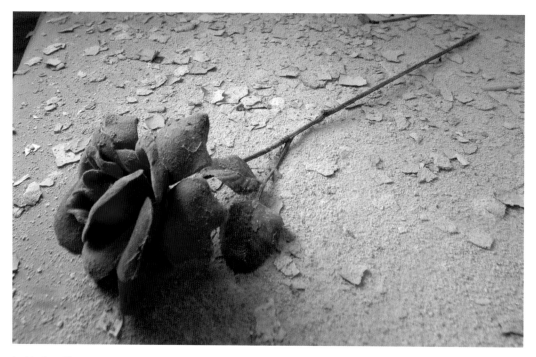

Inside the office, against the far wall, stood a small wooden table covered in flaked plaster and dirt. Upon it lay a brightly colored false flower, filthy but unaffected by the state of the hospital around it. This unexpected bit of symbolism perhaps summarized the whole of the old asylum: a thing timelessly beautiful, dormant, and discarded.

6

SAMUEL R. SMITH INFIRMARY

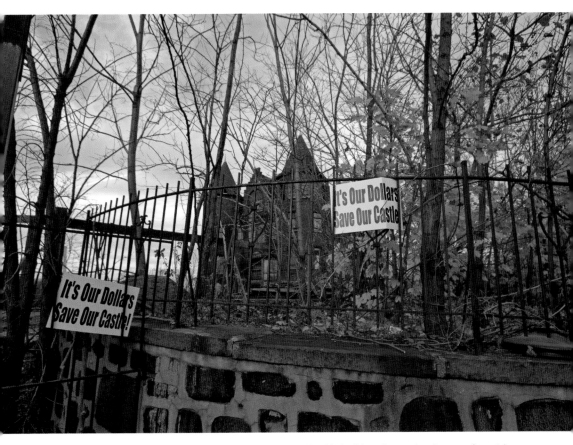

Though the Samuel R. Smith Infirmary of Staten Island, New York, did tend to varying degrees of mental healthcare throughout its years, it never operated as a "true" psychiatric hospital. That said, the old place is worthy of inclusion for a number of reasons, primarily as an example of lost potential. These castle walls fell in early 2012, despite the best efforts of a grassroots group that formed with the hopes of preserving it.

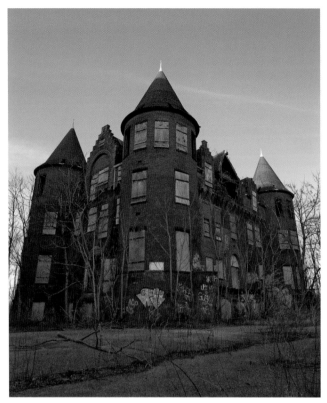

Established by the Richmond County Medical Society in 1861, the Samuel R. Smith Infirmary was the first private hospital built for Staten Island and its residents. In its early years, the Infirmary operated out of a sequence of buildings near the present-day location of the Ferry Terminal. It found a permanent home in 1887, when the Society purchased 6 grassy acres on a hilltop off Castleton Avenue.

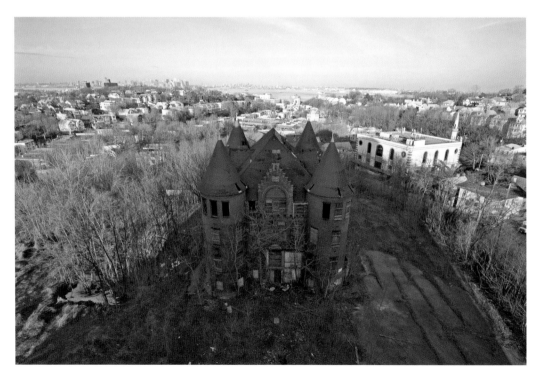

The architect, Alfred E. Barlow, gifted the hospital with a strange and vaguely medieval form, cast in red brick. This was a suiting design choice, however, for what better than a castle to crown an imposing hilltop.

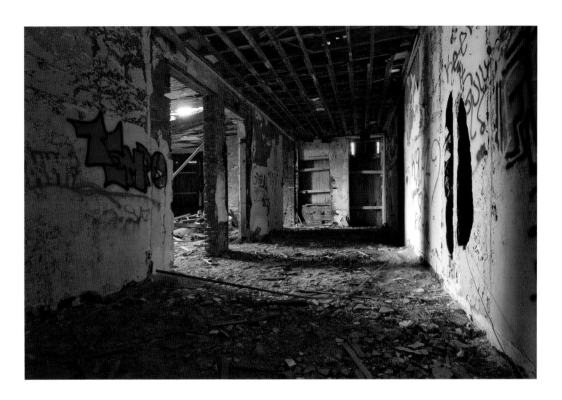

Above: At its opening ceremony, the Infirmary was hailed as the "pride of the island," and it soon went to work serving those in need. Early in its life, the hospital hosted the wounded of the Spanish-American War, when horse-drawn ambulances carried them to its doors in 1898, from the warships Rio Grande, Leona, and Concho in the harbor.

Right: In 1916, the Infirmary was rechristened the Staten Island Hospital. It continued to serve as the primary medical center for the borough until the end of 1979, when it was replaced by a modern, infinitely more ordinary structure on Seaview Avenue in Ocean Breeze.

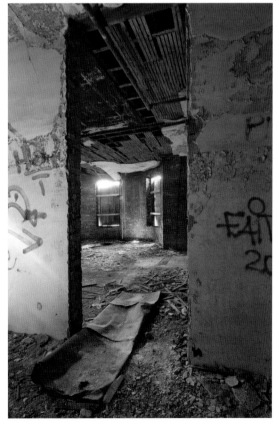

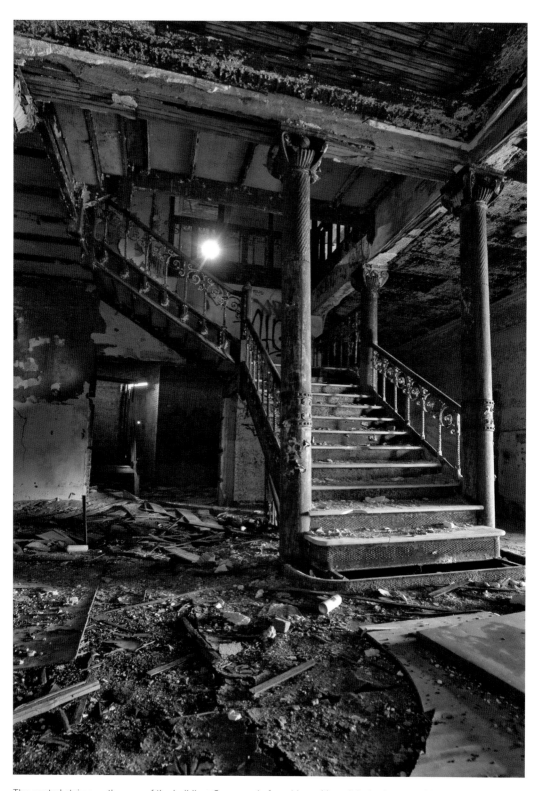

The central staircase, the gem of the building. Composed of marble and iron, it looked on our visit every bit as beautiful as it did when first crafted.

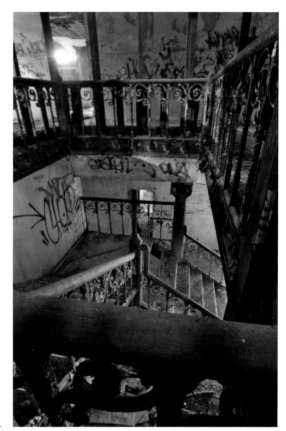

While gaining entry to the hospital was neither easy nor enjoyable, once inside, our company was welcomed with beautiful displays of light, dancing in beams filtering through the branches and decaying walls. It was as if the place was celebrating the presence of people within its walls after an interminable loneliness.

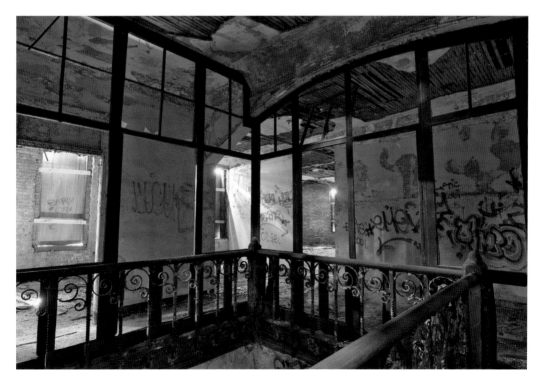

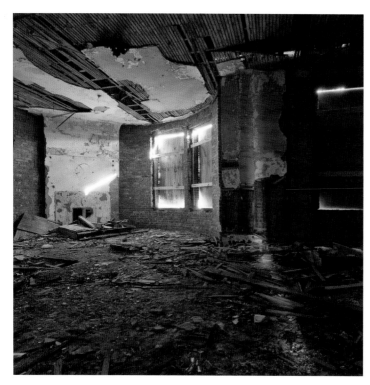

A likely inspiration for the unusual design of the hospital is the then-modern New York Cancer Hospital, built in 1885. It was a common belief at the time that rooms without corners prevented the accumulation of germs and helped mitigate the spread of illness, hence the hospital had many cylindrical chambers.

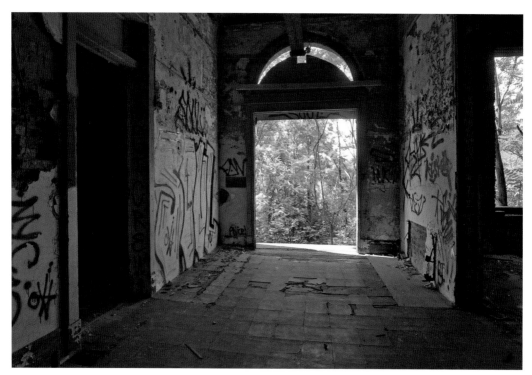

Though standing only several dozen feet in most directions from a roadway or sidewalk, the old hospital had come to be so overgrown with underbrush, trees, and ivy that it all but disappeared from the world outside its fenced hilltop, washed over and dissolved by a newly sprouted urban forest.

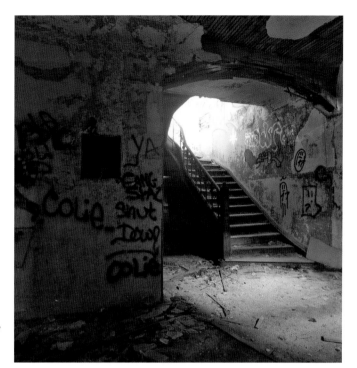

Perhaps it was partially because of the greenery that had come to encompass the old infirmary that it not only faded away from people's daily lives, but from their memories as well.

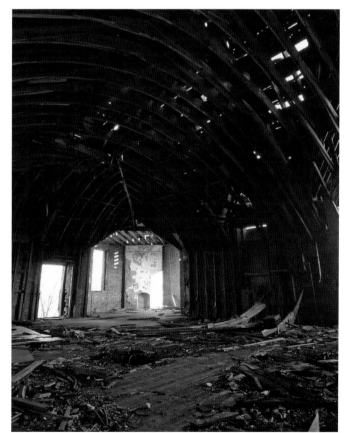

Our ascension through the castle ended at the uppermost floor. What we found there was an immense open space, the exposed beams of its cathedral ceiling looked not unlike that of a ribcage and created in us the uneasy feeling of being trapped in the stomach of a gargantuan, moldering whale.

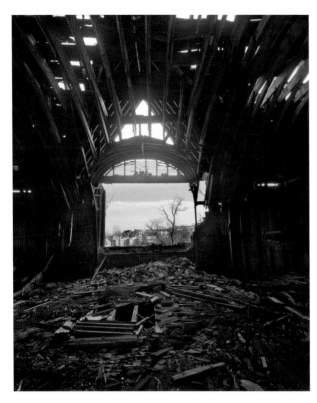

Since its closure, the old hospital sat unused and unmaintained. Slowly, this intriguing piece of architecture and notable piece of Staten Island history was allowed to rot away right under the noses of hundreds of thousands of people, many of whom were born within its walls.

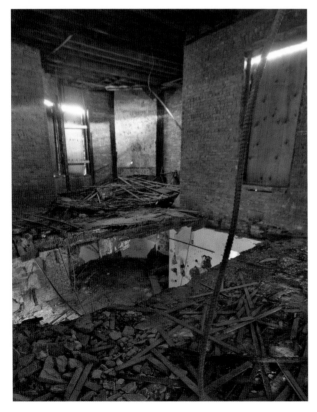

By the time anyone had come to realize what they and the community as a whole were losing to neglect, it was already lost.

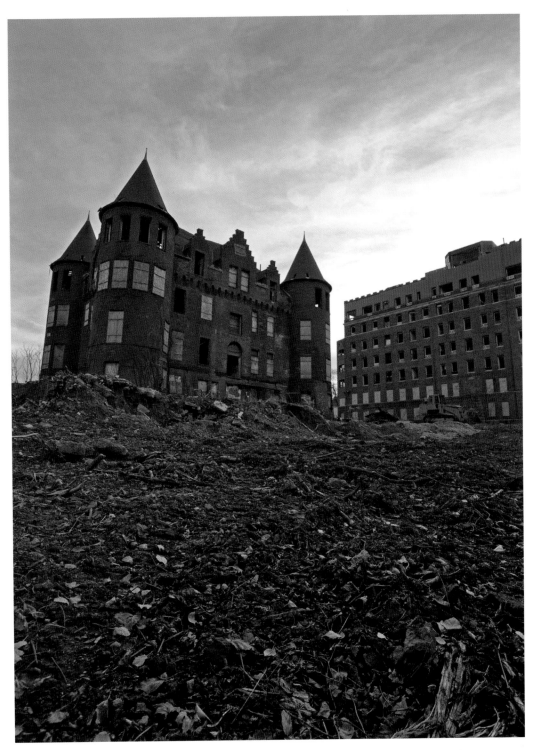

What was once heralded as a great accomplishment had come to be referred to as nothing more than an eyesore. As mentioned earlier, some private groups did organize in an attempt to save the hospital from demolition, and though their intentions were well placed, their actions proved to be a case of too little too late. The castle had peacefully passed away long ago, while slumbering beyond leafy walls of green.

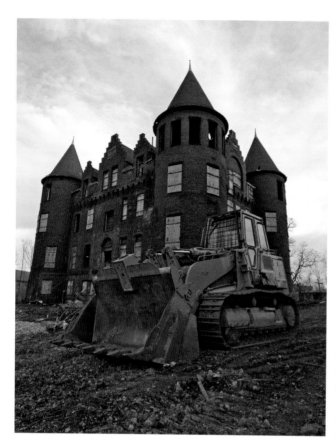

Left and below: In the end, all that remained standing was a decaying shell, one that was far beyond any hope of salvation through reuse, no matter how noble the idea. The forest was cleared, and these castle walls finally fell to the plow on March 5, 2012.

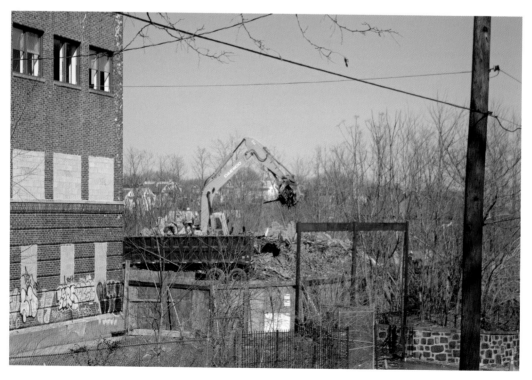

7

EMBREEVILLE STATE HOSPITAL

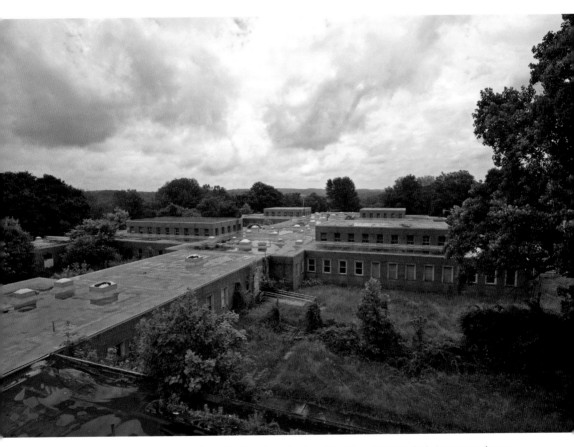

In a rural patch of Pennsylvania can be found a collection of buildings that may look, to a passer-by, as an abandoned school campus. The building exteriors of the Embreeville State Hospital do not outwardly project the image of a psychiatric hospital, and as we learned long ago, first impressions can prove misleading.

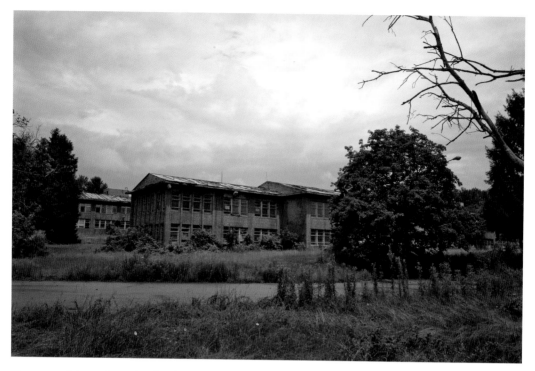

These grounds have changed and evolved in use throughout the years, and as it exists today, the oldest of the structures to stand among the unkempt grasses are of 1930s vintage.

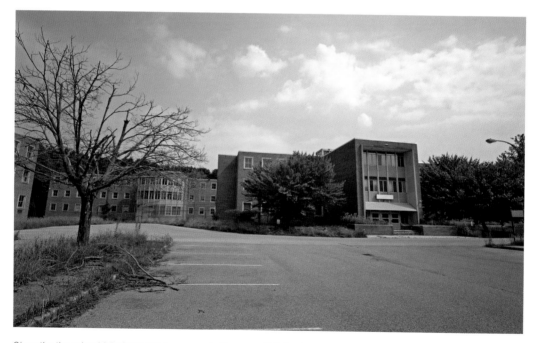

Given the times in which these buildings were built, we see little in the way of the more ornate details that adorn other, often older, state hospital buildings. In their stead, we find mostly flat walls of red brick punctuated by square windows, with flourishes reserved primarily for entryways and bay windows. Still, a style shines through all this, one of a form-follows-function design, which is intriguing in its own right.

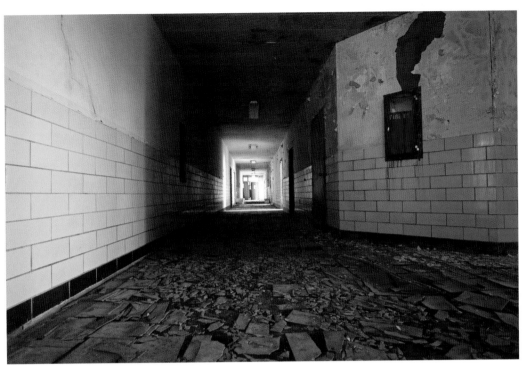

Within the buildings, things were no less rigid; the utilitarian design of the hospital was highly focused and rarely deviated.

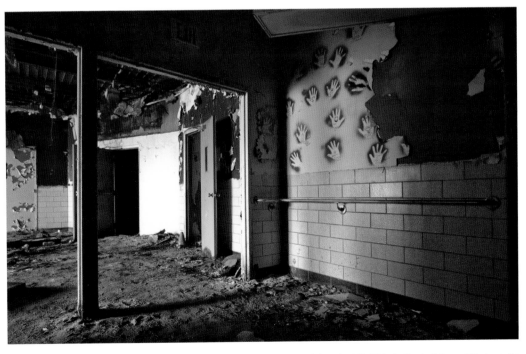

Angular corners and flat walls frame reminders of past lives, and though at first blush, the buildings of Embreeville may seem less interesting than the more grand designs found elsewhere, their simple looks belie the captivating landscape within.

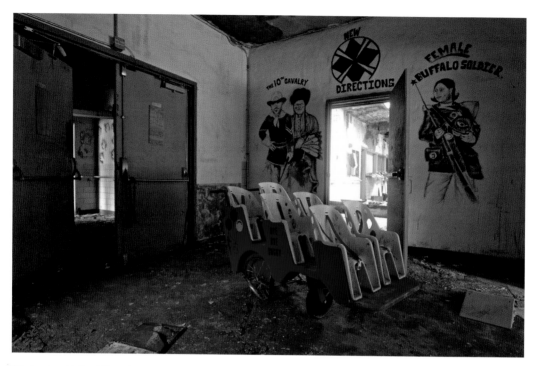

What makes Embreeville unique to us, and why we chose to document it as we have, is that it houses an unusual amount of relics from its past life as a hospital. These items, while perhaps worthless outside these walls in any monetary sense, serve as priceless and poignant relics within these wards. There is a duality of worlds at play: that of what was and that of what is.

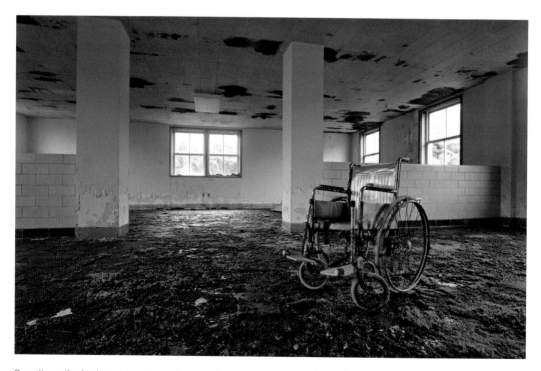

Sometimes the best monument to a place and time is the place itself, left to time.

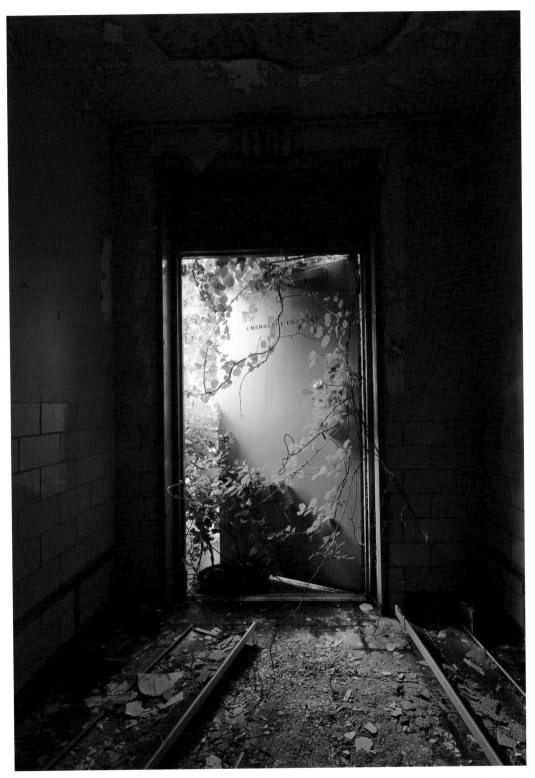

Most of the buildings on this campus have been shuttered since 1980, and in many places, the decades of disuse have become painfully and beautifully, obvious.

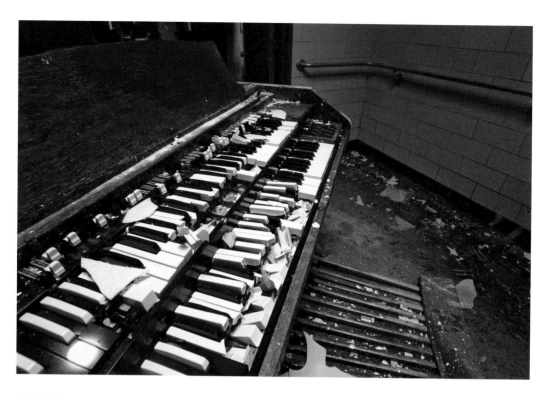

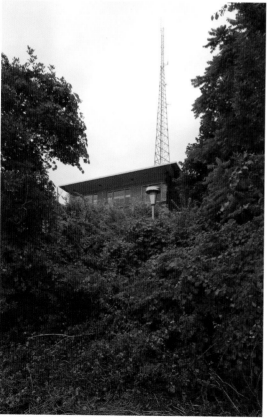

Above: A battered electric organ sits in a hallway below an open skylight. Plant life sprouts between its mangled keys.

Left: Some of the building on the Embreeville campus have become incredibly overgrown. In this case, the front lawn and walkway of this building have been utterly consumed by greenery, much of which stands over 10 feet tall.

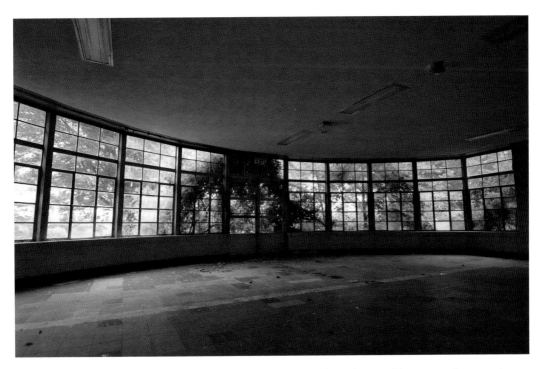

"Stranglehold" is the best way to describe the way in which the ivy and encroaching greenery has come to wrap much of the grounds. In many instances, the overgrowth blots out much of the daylight, creating darkened chambers where sunlight-bathed rooms once were.

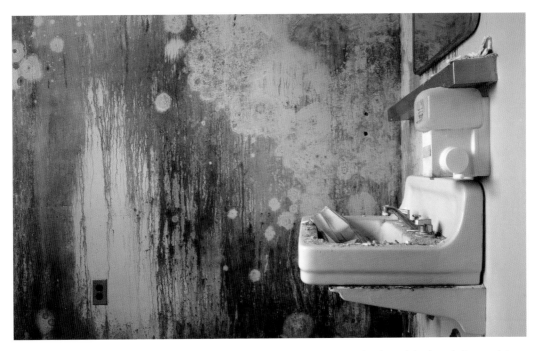

Plant life often found its way inside as well, with branches and vines grasping through broken windows and doors left ajar; however, something altogether different has also laid claim to the old hospital. Molds, neither plant nor animal, is ever-present, feeding upon the softened sheetrock and plaster.

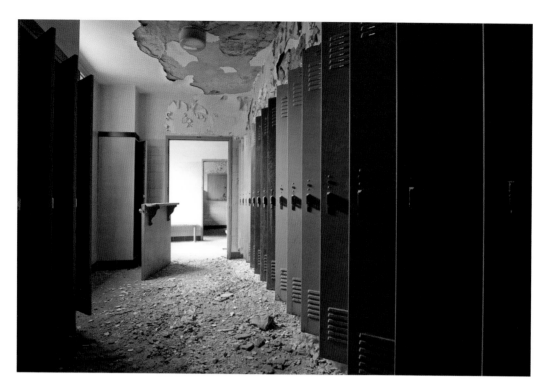

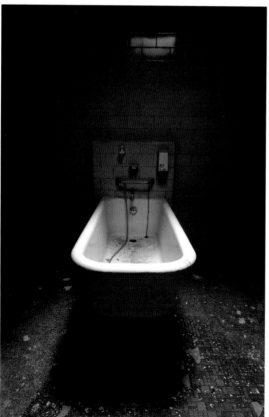

Above: A row of rainbow-hued lockers stand open just outside the old shower room.

Left: In a dark room beyond the lockers can still be found the showers and baths.

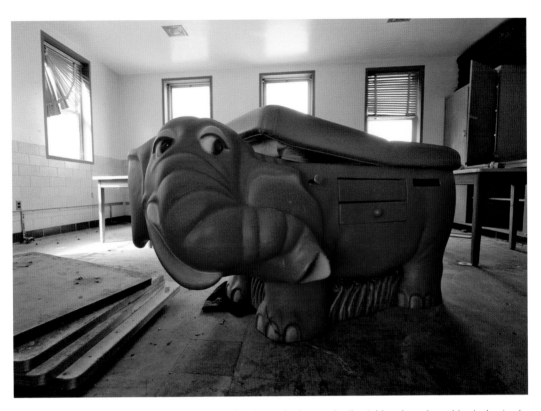

In the pediatric wards roam strange wildlife—large plastic examination tables shaped as whimsical animals, which (supposedly) eased the anxiety of children awaiting a visit from the doctor.

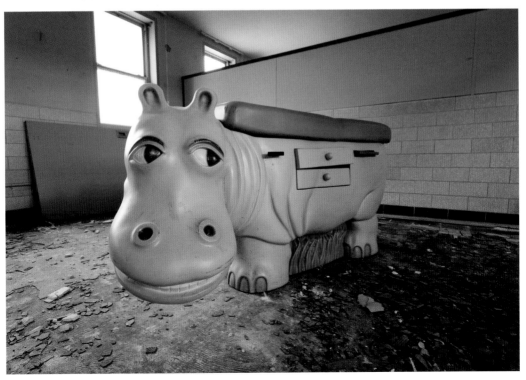

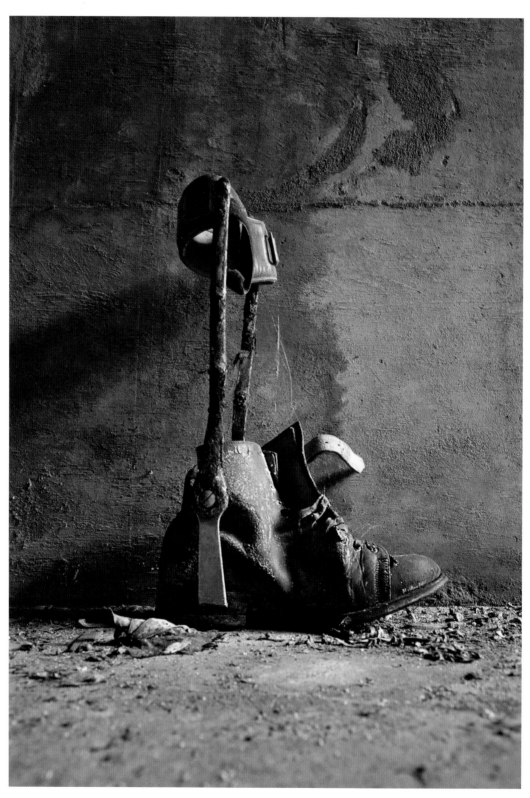

A rusting child's leg brace leans against a concrete wall in the basement. Our last sight as we left the campus.

8

LOST AT SEA

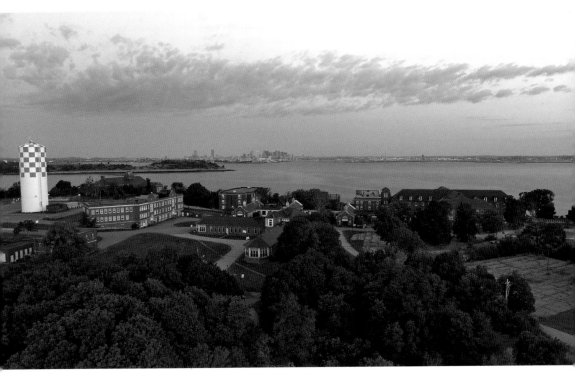

Every place has a tale to tell. Some provide us with insight into things unknown, some evoke empathy for people we never knew, and still others move us with a sense of faith in things unseen. Sometimes, though, the story that sticks with you the most is the one you forged for yourself. In the case of this water-locked asylum, we found ourselves staring at a city-line in the distance, but though we could see the silhouettes of buildings and the glow of lights in the evening, we may as well have been a world away. And in many ways we were.

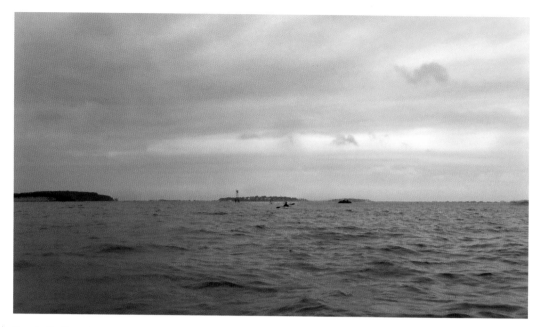

Our destination sat out at sea, well beyond any line of sight from where we currently stood. We were in company this day, our group of four having made a temporary base of operations in a small parking lot. With provisions secured and equipment tie-downs checked one final time, we set to carrying the kayaks down the boat launch. Our plastic vessels were overburdened, and though we had faith in them and ourselves to make the journey across the water, our hearts sank as dark clouds began to churn in the skies above, sucking life from the once-blue until it became a sickly greenish-grey. By the time we had paddled a few miles out from the coast, we were in the midst of a small squall, one that blotted out the shoreline and brought with it swells of more than 2 feet. A turbulence of black water and gray air had enveloped us, which when traveling by lake kayak in the open water with nearly 100 pounds of cargo, quickly becomes an unwelcome test of wills.

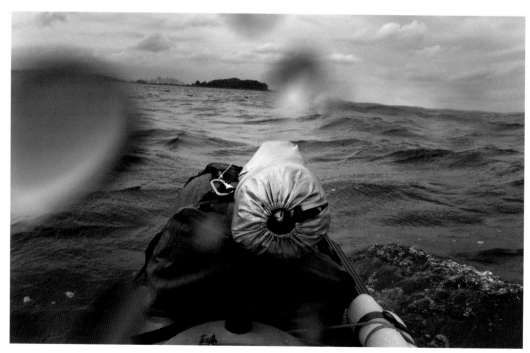

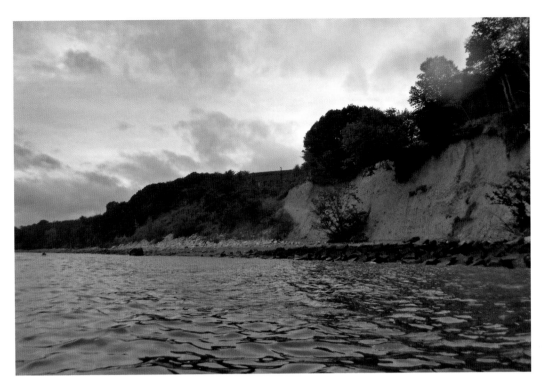

Eventually, the storm waned and we came upon the shoreline of the old hospital grounds. A bluff of stone and thorns greeted us, and just barely peeking out from the top of the rock outcropping, we could see the roof of the old power plant, abandoned long ago, decades before the hospital itself shuttered. This was to be our home for the next two days.

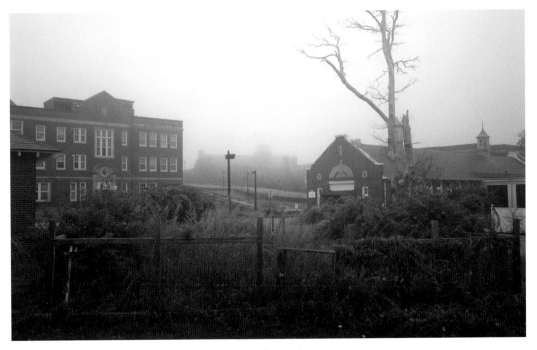

A thick fog welcomed us to the overgrown hospital grounds.

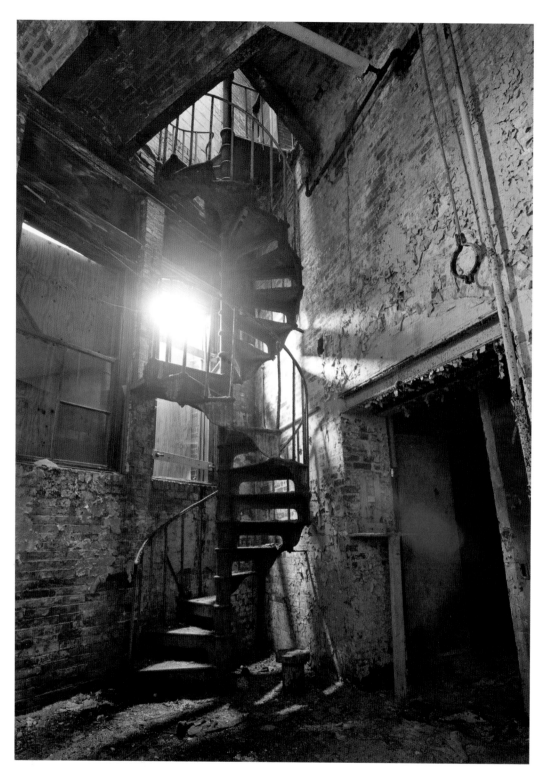

This old spiral staircase of iron was the only access to our campsite on the upper floor of the power plant. Our first night was under thunderous skies and heavy rain—rain which had no difficulty entering through the rotten roofing and partially flooding our home away from home.

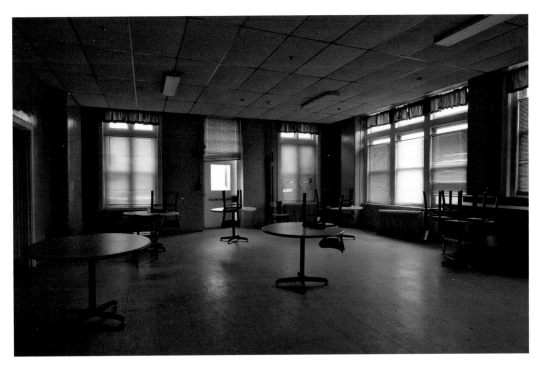

The scenes within the hospital walls were surreal. Having only been shuttered in 2014, and inaccessible with the exception of watercraft, things appeared as if trapped in time. Here, chairs are still stacked upon tables in a small mess hall, as if the morning crew will be in any moment to set them for breakfast.

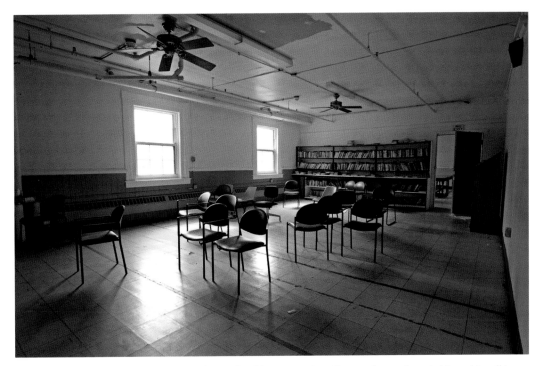

A small lecture room sits in eerie silence. Outside, you can hear the cry of seagulls and chime of far-off buoys in the harbor.

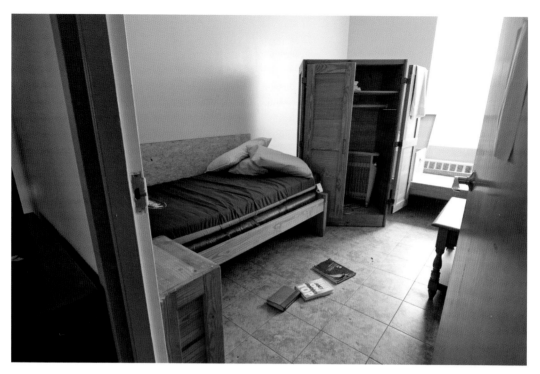

Everywhere, bedrooms lay empty, and in many of them, numerous personal items were left behind—likely the result of the hurried fashion in which the hospital relocated patients in the final days of operation. Without mainland access, once abandoned, these personal effects would prove impossible to return to and retrieve. As they sit today, they paint a picture of the last lives to call this place home.

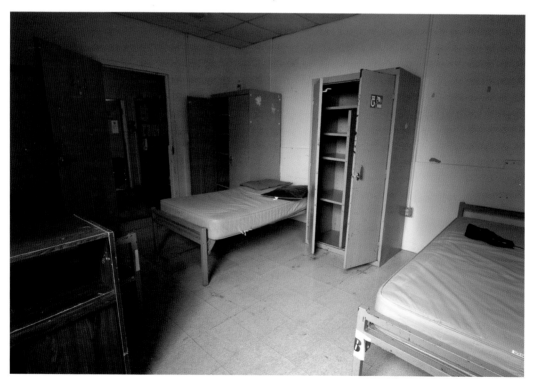

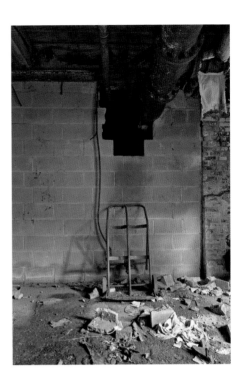

The polished floors of the 1940s era hospital hide away secrets. Down below, in the tunnels that run the grounds, you may find yourself coming upon an out-of-place wall of cinder-block. High upon its face, several blocks are missing, and in their stead is a void of pitch-black darkness. This is a threshold, a concrete dividing line between "now" and "then."

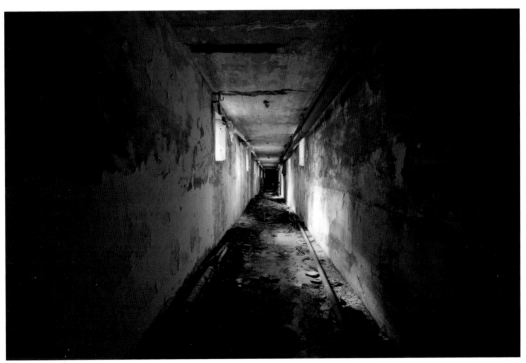

Upon passing through that breach, the truth of the hospital becomes more clear: the chambers and halls above sit upon the bones of something far older. Long ago, an asylum stood on this island, a campus that, in the 1940s, was razed and replaced by what you now find topside. Not all was lost, though; the modern hospital sits on many of the original foundations and tunnel systems of what was there before, and what they did not remove was sealed away behind the cinder-block wall. Here, the past dwells in darkness.

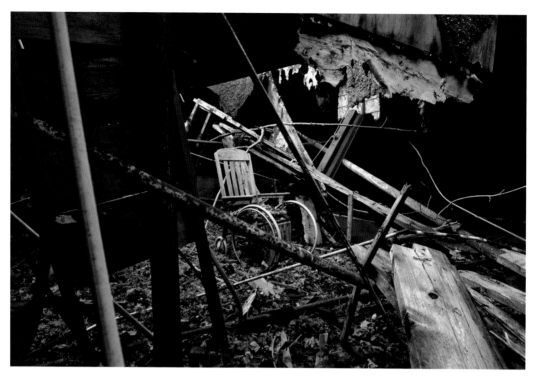

The darkness here is punctuated by swaths of daylight that pours in through collapses where structures and supports above have given away to the forest that now grows above.

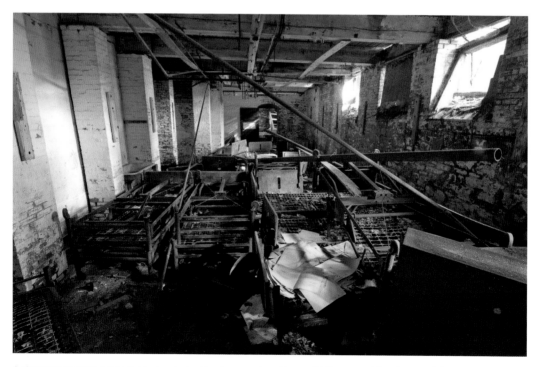

A chamber of antique hospital beds, stacked in storage, placed here a lifetime ago at the closure of the hospital, which once stood on these grounds.

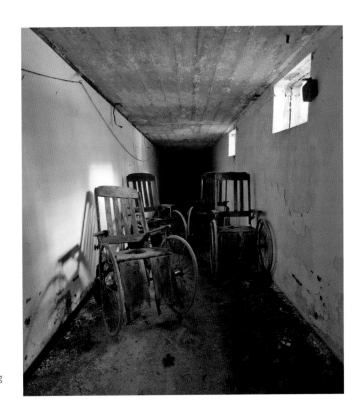

Rotting wooden wheelchairs congregate in a hallway leading into a shadowy abyss.

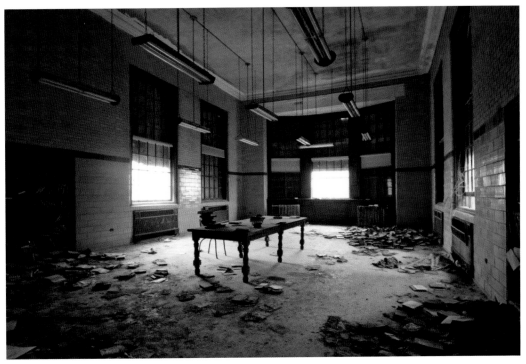

Decay has also set in above ground, on the abandoned structures that dot the outer edges of the grounds. Here, a library crumbles away, much as the ocean beyond slowly erodes away the rocky bluff of the island upon which it stands.

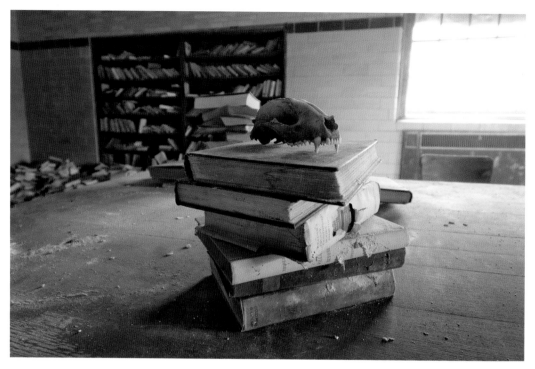

There is a parallel to note between the books rotting away, taking the knowledge contained within them as they turn to dirt, and the similarly decomposing asylum that surrounds them. Once these places succumb to the elements and leave us, they take with them the stories and lessons contained within their walls.

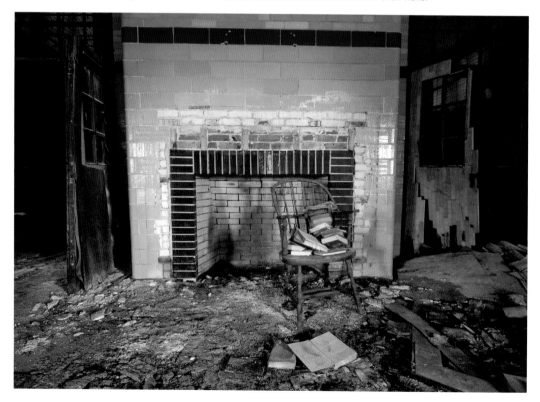

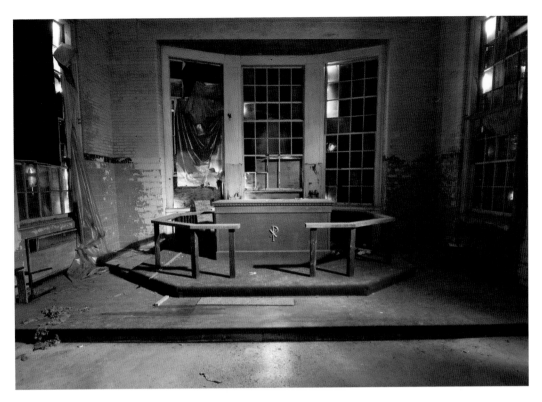

A small chapel, godforsaken.

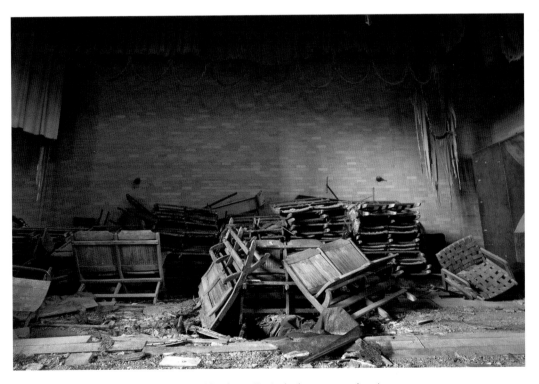

Rows of auditorium seats folded and haphazardly stacked upon a sagging stage.

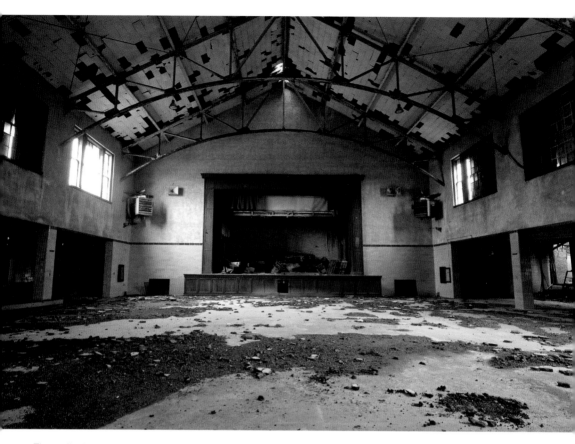

The auditorium, hosting one perpetual final performance as the stage and chamber that houses it slowly return to the earth. Played out to a backing track of the sea forever breaking upon the nearby shoreline.

9

ROCKLAND PSYCHIATRIC HOSPITAL

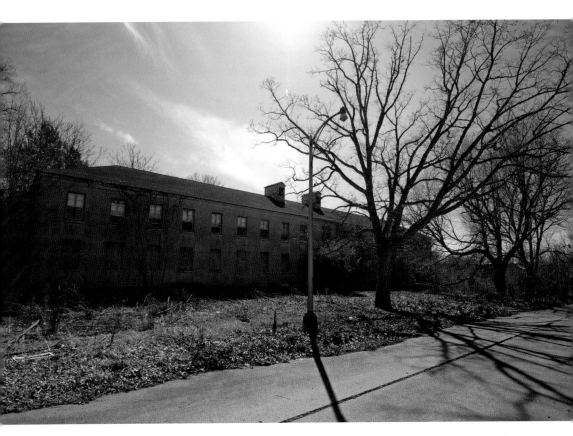

In a point worth noting, a bulk of this campus is being demolished as we write these very pages, and will not exist by the time you are reading this. Long ago, though, things were much different in Rockland County, New York. The quiet morning of May 18, 1927 is splintered as a steam-shovel engine rumbles to life, its slow-moving maws dig deep into the earth. These are the first moments in the creation of New York's latest psychiatric hospital, and what was to go on to be one of the largest mental health complexes in the world: Rockland Psychiatric.

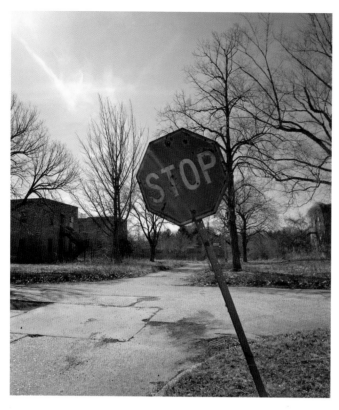

Operating the steam-shovel was then-Governor Alfred Emanuel Smith, Jr., who offered this quote shortly thereafter: "We need a new state hospital at least every three years to keep up with the growth in the number of the committed insane.... The state hospitals are today overcrowded about 30 percent, and the census is growing so rapidly that we can't catch up." Countless more pieces of construction equipment flowed through the property following that day, and together they slowly shaped some 600 acres into a sprawling mental health complex. Like many state-run facilities of this era, it housed its own power plant, and a farm that raised and grew much of its own food. Later on, the campus opened industrial shops crafting mattresses and furniture, primarily operated by the patients who resided there.

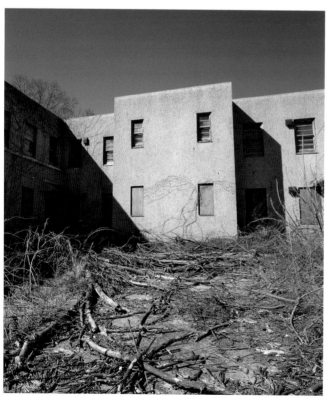

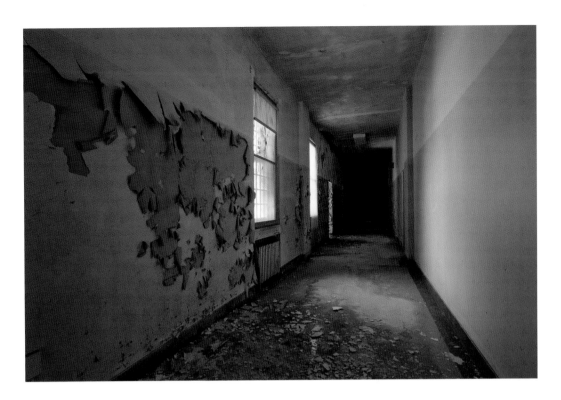

Above: Insulin-shock therapy (a.k.a. insulin coma therapy) was introduced to the facility in 1937. This one-time popular process consists of injecting the patient with large amounts of insulin, enough to put them into a coma. Treatments were often administered on a daily basis for a designated period, at times spanning several weeks in total.

Right: A frozen clock sits high upon a peeling wall, overlooking an office that too seems frozen in time.

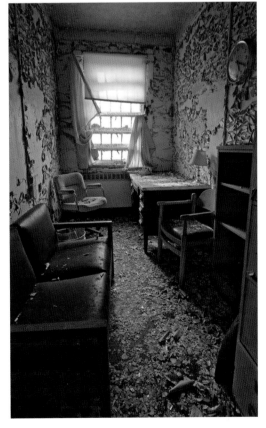

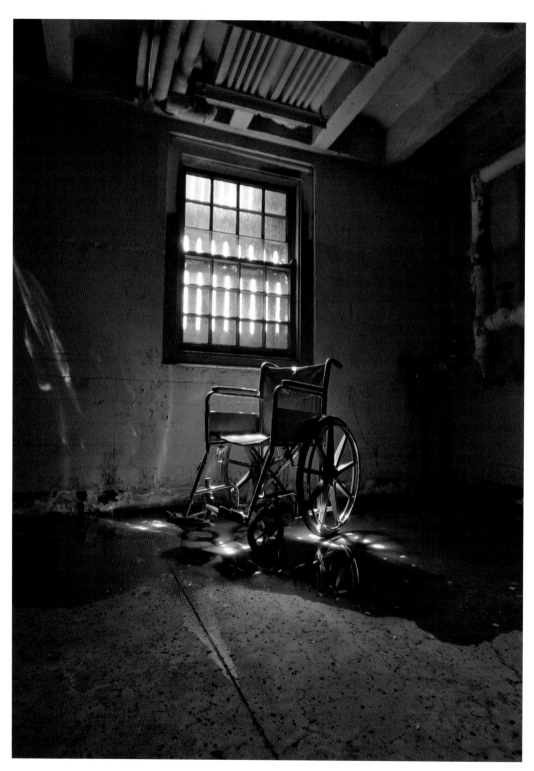

A wheelchair sits in a pool of stagnant water below a basement window while the wards on the floors above it buckle, crack, and crumble. During its day, this massive complex was hailed as one of the nation's best-planned mental health centers.

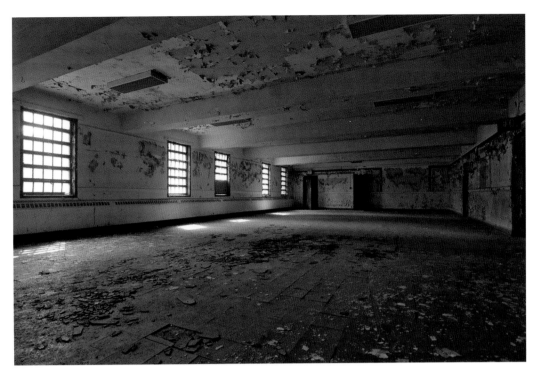

Though the acclaimed facility's prosperous beginnings were thought to have indicated a bright future, within its first decade, the hospital had fallen victim to the same blight that was affecting many other mental health institutions across the nation: severe overcrowding.

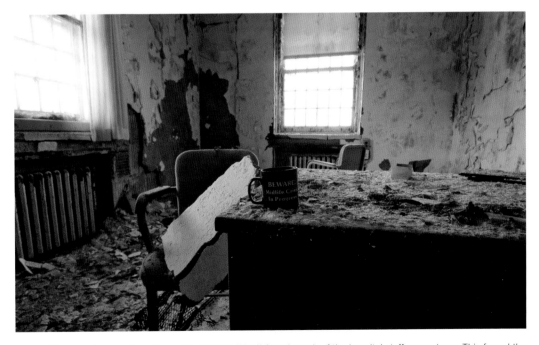

To exacerbate matters, the drafts of World War II found much of the hospital staff away at war. This forced the center to seek out new crewmembers as quickly as possible. Due to this, many of the personnel here were undertrained and terribly unqualified for the tasks asked of them.

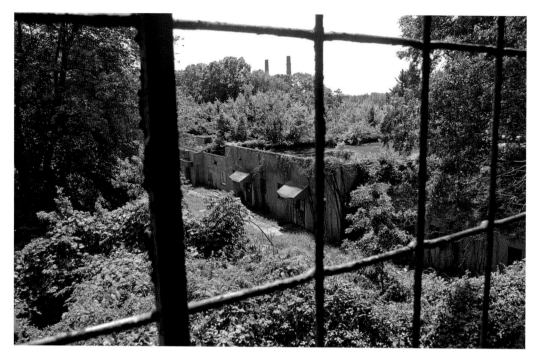

During our visit, Rockland Psychiatric existed in a strange state, a limbo of sorts, operating almost exclusively out of new modern buildings—which tower stories above the old campus—and original buildings—which had been left forgotten and severely overgrown. This mid-summer view from within an enclosed patient porch shows just how wild some of the campus had become.

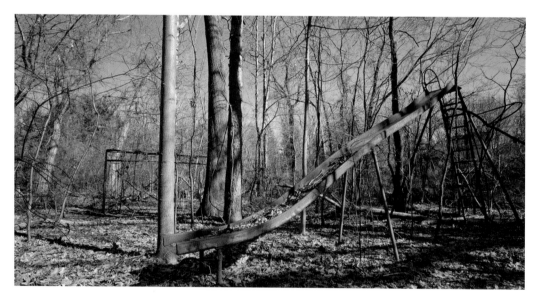

A playground rusts away in the woods, wrapped in vines, thorns, and neglect. As a molting insect discards its shell as it grows, this hospital has shed off its former campus *in lieu* of impressive towers that gleam with all the promises and majesty of modern medicine—just as the old campus once did. Perhaps it was wished that nature simply reclaim these old wards, and with them, the history contained within. Like many other forgotten asylums across our nation, the discarded buildings of Rockland Psychiatric were a physical representation of America's great shift in mental healthcare, for better and worse.

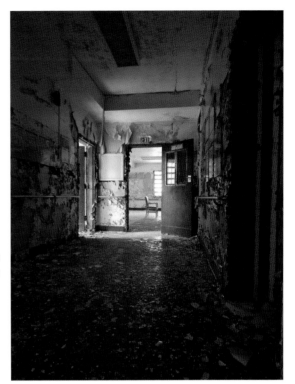

Further compounding the hardships that the hospital was already facing in the late 1930s and early 1940s with regards to limited staff, the asylum also quickly came to lack the physical space to properly house and care for the all the patients now living there. This found beds being placed in hallways and dayrooms, creating a breeding ground for the spread of illness and infection.

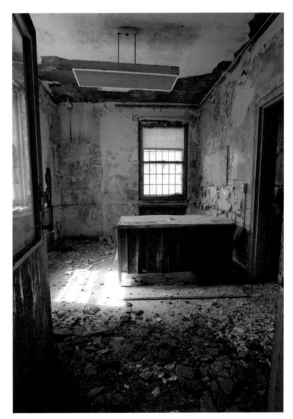

A desk rots away in a long-shuttered office. The year 1959 marked the peak for admittance to the hospital, pushing the total patient population to over 7,000. To put that into a proper perspective, it meant there was just one psychologist for every 300 patients.

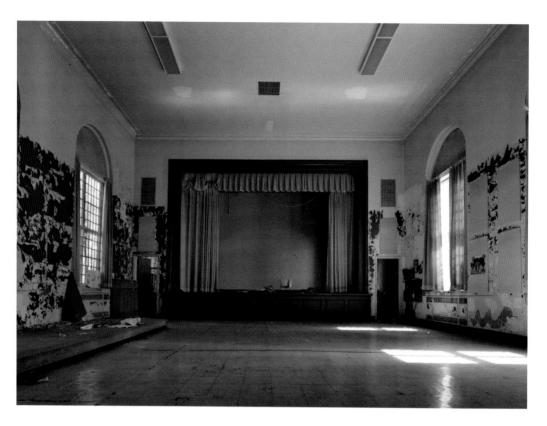

Above: Quiet and stillness sit heavily in the air within a former amusement hall. The building that housed this stage was disused by the hospital long ago, but later became repurposed as a childcare center—for a time.

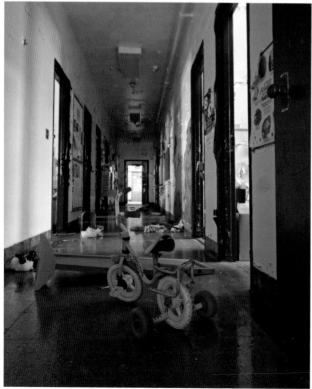

Left: In the corridors beyond the amusement hall, children's toys scatter the floors.

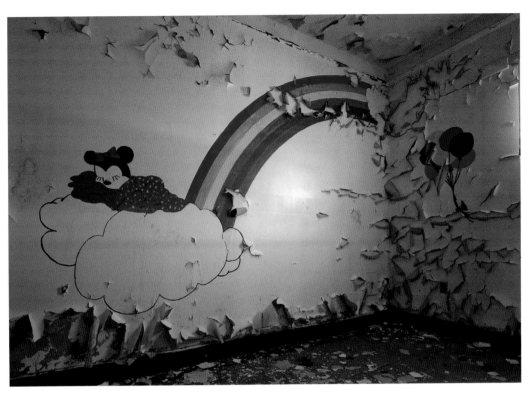

Above and below: Perhaps the most powerful reminders of what once existed here were the murals, which became cracked and distorted echoes of what they once were. Once-cheerful scenes laid upon the very walls, undone by the workings of time.

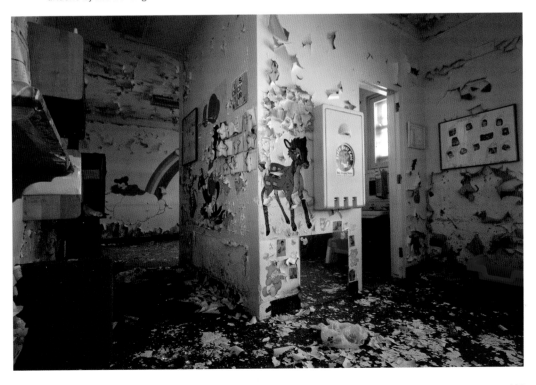

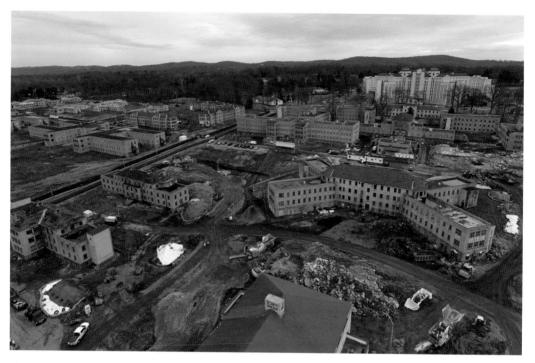

This aerial photo by our close friend "GlideByJJ"/Jody Johnson, taken during the early phases of demolition, shows just how large the old Rockland campus used to be. In the upper-right of the frame can be seen the modern and still-operational hospital that came to replace the old, cottage style wards that now fall away under its gaze.

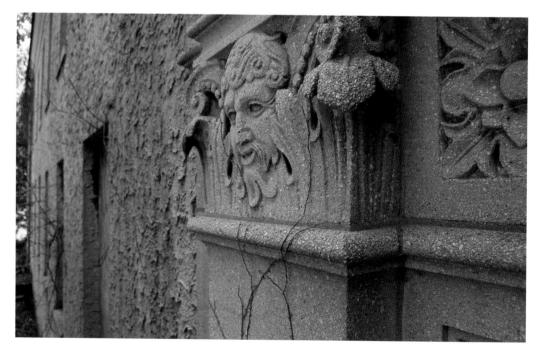

Much like how the forest slowly hid away these old buildings, so too can the passing of time fog over our memories of even the most tragic events. To forget what happened here would be the single greatest disservice we could inflict upon those who lived it.

10

BUFFALO REBORN

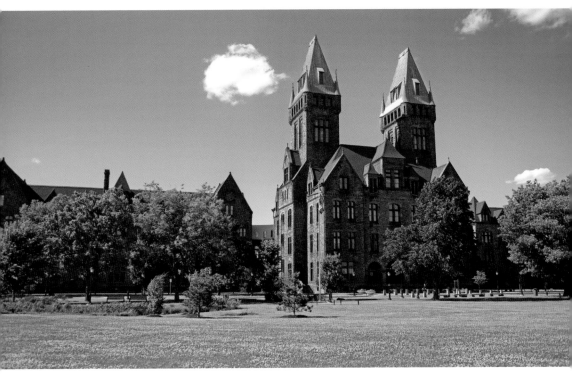

With this page, we enter the conclusion of this book, and like any book worthy of a reader's time, we have chosen to conclude with a moral to our story—a universal truth that rings well beyond the subject matter of abandoned asylums: painful histories are the ones most easily forgotten. Even if only for that reason, we as a society need to think hard upon what we are doing with our nation's disused asylum buildings. If we remove them from our landscape, we too remove them and their stories from our minds. The generations who follow us will never grasp what came before if they cannot, see, feel, and listen to the buildings for themselves. Luckily, there now exist brilliant examples of what can be done with these places often cited as too large or historically complex to adaptively reuse, and a glowing example can be found in the city of Buffalo, New York.

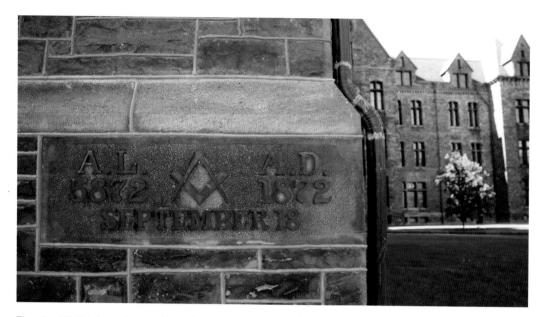

The city of Buffalo is a unique and historic city in and of itself, but what sets it apart from many others is that, within its boundaries, stands a building of great national importance. A gem that has spent decades tarnished, but is now finally shining again: the Richardson Olmsted Complex, or as it was once known in a past life, the Buffalo State Asylum for the Insane.

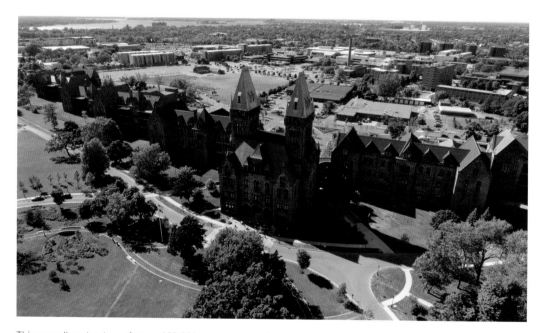

This sprawling structure of some 463,000 square feet had stood mostly empty and disused since 1974, and completely abandoned since 1994. In the years thereafter, its darkened form stood as a vacant and imposing white elephant, a ghost of the city's past. Demolition became a very real possibility, one that was taken to court to keep from occurring. Today, though, things are much different. The darkness has been lifted and the building once again shines. Life has returned to its halls thanks to the dedicated work of the Richardson Center Corporation and now the Hotel Henry, which opened in April 2017, the first tenant in the multi-phase redevelopment plan for the beautiful old campus.

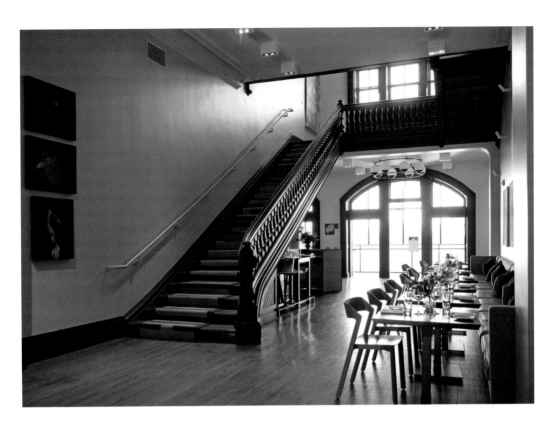

The Hotel Henry takes up about one-third of the former hospital, including the entirety of the iconic central building and the first two wings on either side; beyond, the vacant hospital wards still sit silent and empty, awaiting eventual reuse. The fashion in which the modern hotel melds itself with the historic hospital is incredible to behold. Here, the iconic original master stairwell has been cleaned of its decades of dust, refinished, and once again welcomes visitors as the centerpiece of the hotel lobby.

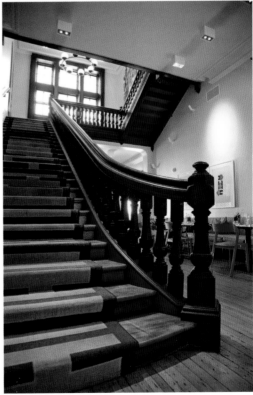

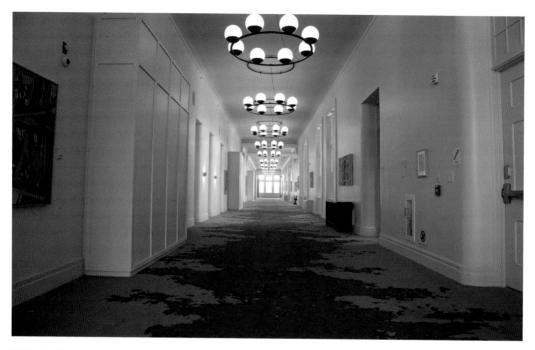

Within the hotel, old meets new in unexpected ways. Old ward corridors now house the hotel's guestrooms, and though modernized, it still retains much of the century and a half of historic character that the walls have been embodied with.

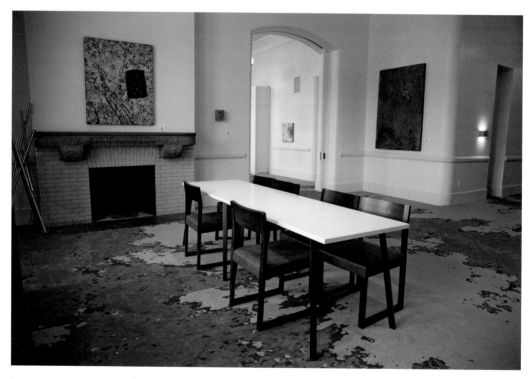

Here, a former common area for patients has been transformed into a sitting area for guests. The original fireplace and carved mantel remain, again allowing the past to echo through to the present day.

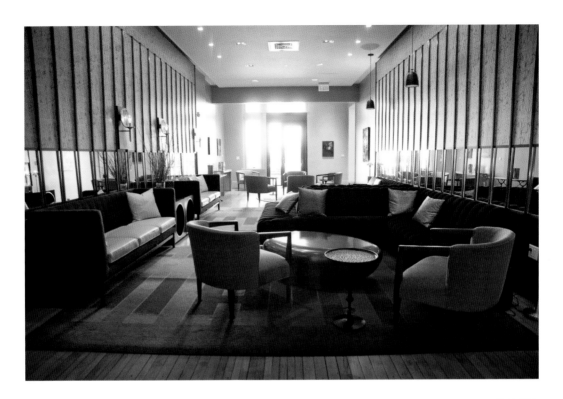

Above: The hotel lounge, occupying a space that once housed administrative offices. Time and time again, preservation efforts regarding asylum structures are met with uninformed opponents who, among other equally invalid arguments, often debate that the rehabilitation of such a structure will not prove commercially viable, using tired lines such as "no one will want to spend their time or money in a former psychiatric hospital." Jessica Mancini, the Digital Marketing Manager at Hotel Henry, paints quite the opposite picture: "The public was very excited, we sold out an entire month before the hotel even opened."

Right: Jessica continued: "We look for ways to invite the public in for free, so they can experience the building. The first thing we did was curate a permanent collection of art, all from western-New York artists.... The first art opening we had, we expected 250 people to show up, and we got two thousand, and I think that speaks to the public's want to see this space." Pictured here is a corridor gallery space, an area of the hotel that retains the original hospital tile-work.

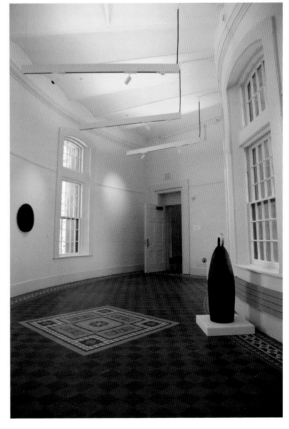

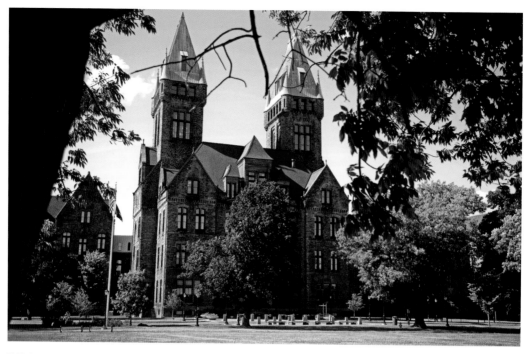

Utilizing the former asylum as a hotel allows visitors to better understand that these historic asylums were not built as the haunting places they are all too often portrayed as in films or sensationalized as in television "reality" shows. At their construction, these campuses were raised as luxurious resorts that were to provide a place for the place-less. Magnificent castles built for the care of those who, many of which, could not even say "thank you."

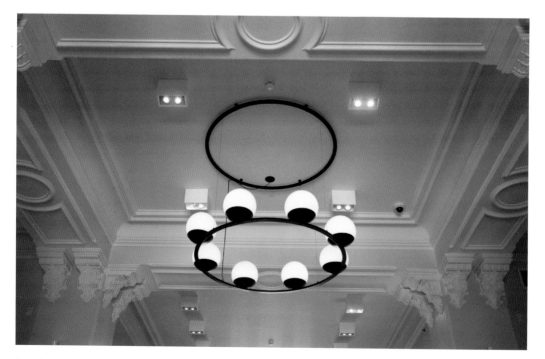

Attention to detail was paid in equal measure both outside and inside, as shown in this detail shot of Hotel Henry's lobby. Modern light fixtures punctuate antique moldings and woodwork.

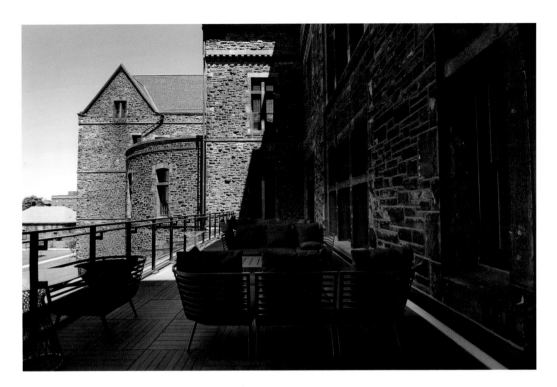

Above: An outdoor sitting area perched upon the second floor of the rear entrance of the former hospital, with views of the curved corridors that lead out toward the tiered wards, which stretch outward into the distance. A space purposely designed to allow one to simply sit and admire their surroundings.

Right: A flower arrangement in an alcove, a scene that is just at place today in a modern hotel as it would have been well over a century ago when this was a thriving psychiatric hospital. It was common practice to have an abundance of flower arrangements throughout the hospital in an effort to soothe patients through picturesque settings. "Beauty as therapy" was the common phrase.

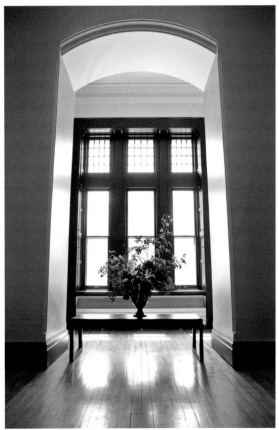

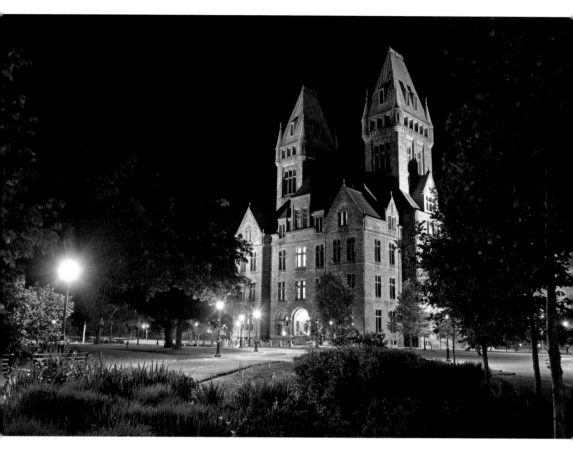

The Richard Olmsted complex, and the other hospitals across the country that share in its design, are arguably some of the most noble and compassionate constructions our nation has ever created. The thought that they can so easily be thrown aside, abandoned to rot, viewed as haunted houses unworthy of preservation speaks volumes about the stigmas that are still attached to mental illness.

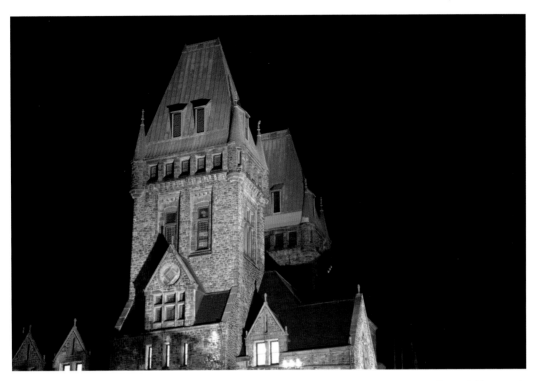

With such a successful example as Hotel Henry to look to, we have no excuse not to seek out viable reuse in every instance where demolition of a historic asylum is presented. We cannot bury our past, no matter how large the bulldozer. We must embrace our collective history, all of it, no matter how dark it can be at times. Celebrate it, cast a light upon it so bright that it may never be forgotten.

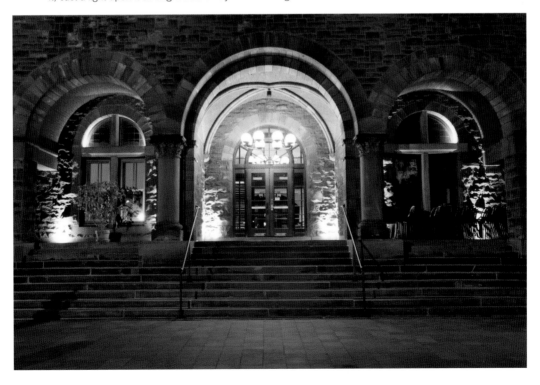

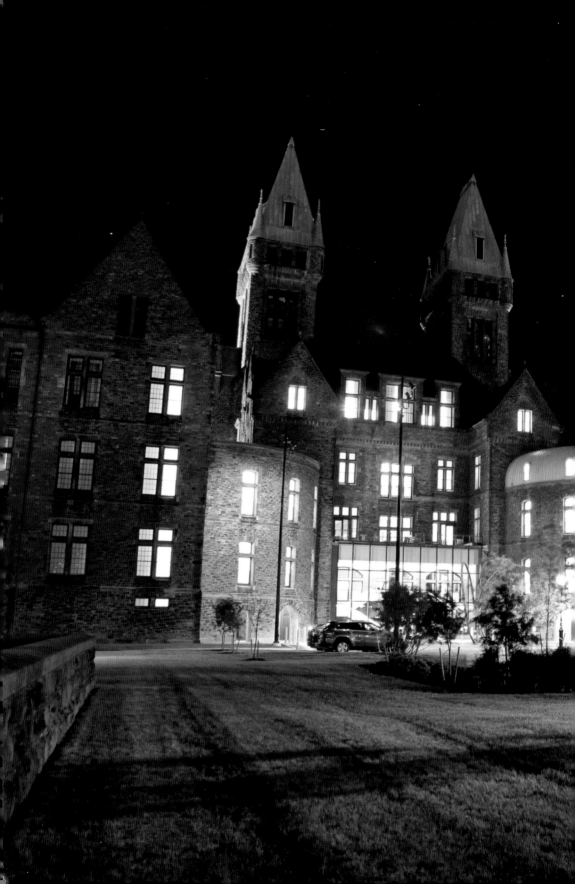

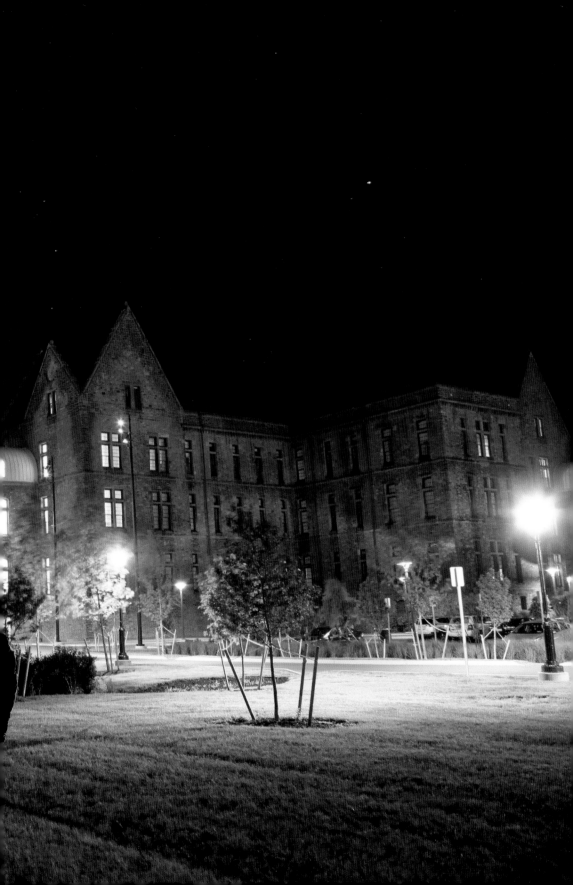

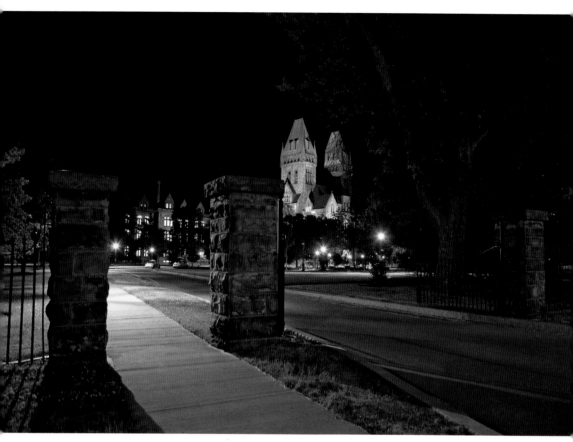

The old hospital gates—originally built as a welcoming entryway to a public park and gardens—eventually, through unfortunate events, had come to be seen as a threshold few wished to cross. Today, the grounds are once again celebrated, and the building once again warmly welcomes you into its presence. Even after dark, there is an immense beauty here, but it differs than that of what is found in the day. After the sun has set, and a deep quiet drapes the campus, one can sit alone on the cool grass and ponder the stone facade staring back at you. And so it is, a beautiful building nearly lost, now lives again as a place of purpose and insight for Buffalo to be proud of. For us all to be proud of. Though the complex still has a way to travel on its road to rehabilitation, the Hotel Henry has returned life to its heart. It beats now.

Previous page: The Richardson Olmsted Complex, with the Hotel Henry at the center, shines as a beacon. Far beyond the reaches of the literal radiance, which has now returned to these old halls, there is a light of opportunity—of leading by example, which in turn ignites a light within each person who sees it.

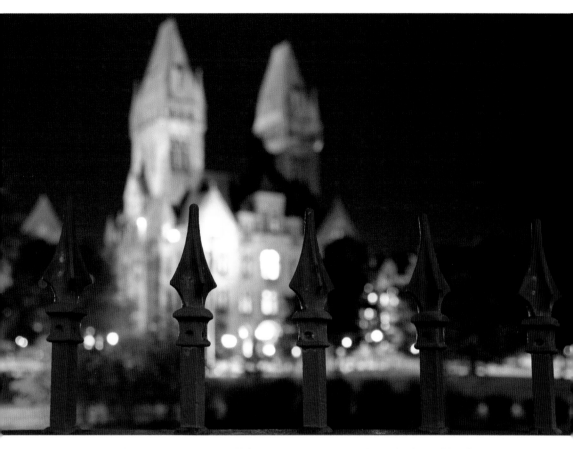

"The tapestry of history has no point at which you can cut it and leave the design intelligible," Dorothea Dix.